The Neurosciences and Behaviour

An Introduction

Second Edition

The Neurosciences and Behaviour

An Introduction

Second Edition

Dale M. Atrens
University of Sydney

Ian S. Curthoys
University of Sydney

ACADEMIC PRESS
A Subsidiary of Harcourt Brace Jovanovich, Publishers
Sydney New York London
Paris San Diego San Francisco São Paulo Tokyo Toronto

Printed in Australia

National Library of Australia Cataloguing-in-Publication Data

---

Atrens, Dale M. (Dale Michael), 1941–.
    The neurosciences and behaviour: an introduction.

    2nd ed.
    Previous ed.: Marrickville, N.S.W.: Science Press, 1978.
    Includes bibliographies and index.
    ISBN 0 12 066850 5.

    1. Neurology. I. Curthoys, Ian S. (Ian Stewart), 1942–.
    II. Title.

616.8

Library of Congress Catalog Card Number: 81-67866

Preface

It has been said that the brain is the last great frontier of research. However, the questions which attract the greatest interest usually do not concern the brain as such. They are more often concerned with behaviour, used in its broadest sense to include sensation, thinking and feeling, as well as actual motor activity.

The widespread and rapidly growing interest in the neurosciences has developed largely because the brain provides a potential key to our understanding of what we do and why we do it. This book has been designed to communicate simply some essentials of the neurosciences with special reference to the problems of how we think, feel and behave. Although most research in the neurosciences is carried out with laboratory animals, we have tried to keep a constant association with the problems of human behaviour.

Little space has been given to the historical development of the material. To paraphrase Ebbinghaus, "the neurosciences have a long past but only a short history". Some fields of research in the neurosciences change relatively slowly, but others have developed only recently and are changing rapidly. For example, many important concepts of anatomy, physiology, sensation and perception have a clear lineage back into the 19th century. With respect to the biological basis of psychiatry, contemporary concepts and theories have only tenuous relationships with any research before the mid-1950s. The neurosciences are in their infancy, and we feel that we can best contribute to their development not so much by the dissemination of a body of facts alone, but rather by encouraging the asking of more and better questions.

We would like to thank the following for their contributions to this project: Patsy Armati, Dick Bandler, Helen Beh, Makram Girgis, Dick Keesey, George Oliphant, George Paxinos, John Sinden, Peter Wenderoth, Bob Gleeson and our publisher.

Contents

8   Reinforcement Mechanisms

9   Emotions, Sex and Aggression

10   Learning and Memory

1
Neurophysiology

1.1 Introduction

The complex processes we call behaviour — thinking, feeling and doing — are clearly determined by simpler processes. What we perceive when we watch a movie depends on information being received by our eyes, travelling to the brain and being processed. The first half of this book is concerned with describing the simpler processes underlying behaviour. The second half is concerned with how these simpler processes are organized into larger units of behaviour. We start by describing the elements of the nervous system, how they receive and transmit information, and how they are organized in the brain.

Cells are the fundamental units of all living organisms — the building blocks of life. There are several features common to most cells:

- a semi-permeable *membrane* which forms the outer wall of the cell and regulates the exchange of nutrients and waste products, and the movement of some important ions;
- the *cytoplasm*, or cell fluid, which contains water, nutrients and ions;
- the *organelles*, distinctive structures which are the cell's machinery for making proteins and which assist the cell's utilization of energy, and
- a *nucleus* which regulates cell reproduction.

We are primarily interested in how organisms interact with their environment (behaviour). We thus concentrate on those cells that are specialized to fulfil this function — the cells of the nervous system. The membranes of nerve cells have evolved two important characteristics which underlie their unique role — they

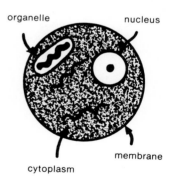

Schematic characteristics of a typical cell.

Cells of the nervous system are specialized to receive and conduct information.

are "excitable", and are able to transmit their "excitation" to other cells.

In the average human brain there are about 10^{12} nerve cells. By way of example, a cylindrical piece of brain 1 mm in diameter and 2 mm in length would contain approximately 35,000 nerve cells.

The nervous system also contains several varieties of satellite cells. One type of satellite cell is the glial cell. Glial cells outnumber nerve cells by 10 to 1 and have been thought of traditionally as structural elements. However, recent information suggests that glial cells may also be involved in nerve cell growth and nutrition, and in the modulation of nerve cell excitability.

There are two types of nerve cells — receptors and neurons.

Interaction with the environment depends on three cell types — receptors, effectors and neurons. There are many similarities between receptors and neurons, and the term "nerve cell" will be used to refer to both these types of cell.

Receptors detect changes in the environment. Effectors actively alter the environment.

Receptors. Receptor cells are especially sensitive to changes in the internal or external environment. They convert energy from one form (such as light) into energy which can be used by the nervous system. While most receptor cells are specialized to detect one particular form of energy, the specialization is not complete. For example, photoreceptors, which normally respond to light, can respond to other forms of energy, such as mechanical pressure. Gently pressing your eyeball with your finger will produce a sensation of light. The physiological implications of such illusions are discussed in section 5.1.

Some receptors, such as those for warmth, touch and pain, are distributed over the entire body surface. However others, such as those of the eyes and ears, are found in discrete groups called sense organs.

Effectors. While receptors function specifically to receive stimulation, they cannot actively affect the environment. This is the function of muscle and gland cells, which are collectively called effector cells. Muscle cells respond by contracting, while gland cells respond by secreting certain substances. In the simplest of systems, information received by a receptor passes directly to an effector cell.

Effector cells, like nerve cells, are excitable. However, unlike nerve cells, they do not convey their excitation to other cells. Thus, strictly speaking, effectors are not part of the nervous system. They are the "executive arm" of the nervous system.

Nerve cells are called neurons. Neurons conduct information and do not reproduce themselves.

Neurons. Generally the information detected by receptors is transmitted to the effectors by neurons. These intervening cells are specialized to conduct and process information and to signal the appropriate responses.

Unlike most other cells in the body, neurons cannot reproduce themselves. Thus at birth the human possesses all the nerve cells it will ever have. In the early months of life, these cells grow in size and complexity, but thereafter they start dying at an estimated rate of 1000 per day. The progressive loss of neurons may be a major factor contributing to the intellectual deterioration (senility) of old age.

Further, nerve cells consume a large amount of energy. Although the brain represents only about 2.5% of our total body weight, it accounts for 25% of our body's oxygen consumption. Because of their voracious appetite, nerve cells may be damaged by even short periods of oxygen deprivation. Any interruption of blood supply to the brain, for example by a blood clot or burst blood vessel, will kill the neurons in that part of the brain by oxygen deprivation. A naturally occurring brain lesion such as this is called a *stroke*. In severe strokes, large areas of the brain are deprived of oxygen, and the loss of function resulting from neuron-loss is both immediate and obvious.

In cases of small but recurrent neural loss, the loss of function becomes apparent only over a period of years. Boxers suffer regular bruising of the brain, and in some this is later manifest in patterns of movement and speech disorders. Such persons are commonly referred to as being "punch drunk". Arteriosclerosis, which causes oxygen deprivation by the progressive narrowing of cerebral arteries, also produces a slow and progressive loss of neurons; as does oxygen deprivation at birth.

There are other less obvious cases of neuron death due to lack of oxygen. Brain tumours are rarely due to changes or altered growth in nerve cells themselves. Usually, brain tumours are due to changes or altered growth in glial cells. The uncontrolled growth of glial cells displaces nerve cells and leads to increasing pressure of the enlarging brain in the fixed confines of the skull. This increasing pressure can reduce the blood flow and oxygen supply to nerve cells, which eventually die. Another example of neuron damage caused by increasing pressure occurs in lead poisoning. One reason lead destroys neurons is that they take up the lead and swell. Again, swelling of the brain within the fixed skull reduces the oxygen supply and kills the neurons.

Nerve cells require a very stable and special environment in order to function properly. Nutritional and other deficiencies in the environment may give rise to abnormalities of neural function and behaviour. For example, a particular pattern of memory and language disorders — the Wernicke-Korsakoff syndrome — has been shown to be due to brain damage caused by lack of vitamin B_1. Such findings have led to the suggestion that some forms of epilepsy and psychiatric disturbances might be due to inherited or acquired metabolic disorders of the brain.

Nerve cells are also susceptible to certain poisons, particularly during growth of the neuron. Mercury and organic chemicals have given rise to tragic illustrations of the behavioural con-

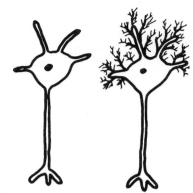

During growth the branches (dendrites) on a neuron increase — in number and complexity.

Neurons are particularly susceptible to lack of oxygen. A stroke is a loss of neurons in the brain due to lack of blood.

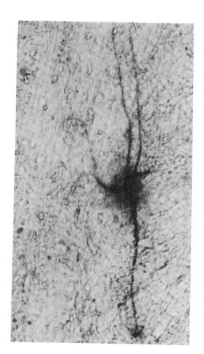

A neuron labelled with the tracer chemical horseradish peroxidase (see 2.1).

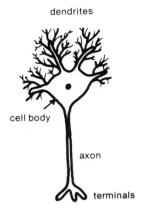

The main structural features of a typical neuron are: dendrites, cell body, axon and terminals.

sequences of neural poisoning (for example, at Minamata Bay in Japan throughout the 1950s).

The following sections consider general features of the often similar structure and function of receptors and neurons.

1.2 Structure of receptors and neurons

A neuron has three main structural features, a *cell-body* or *soma*, an *axon* and a number of *dendrites*. Dendrites are branch-like extensions of the cell-body, the number and arrangement of which vary enormously from neuron to neuron. Generally, the function of dendrites is to carry information to the cell-body. Most receptors and neurons have a special tubular extension of the cell-body — the axon — which, in general, carries information away from the cell-body.

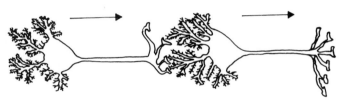

The arrows show the normal direction of information flow within a neuron — from the dendrites to the axon.

Axons vary considerably in both the number of branches or collaterals they make, and in length (the longest axon in man being approximately one metre in length). The greater the number of axon collaterals, the greater the number of cells to which information can be passed. Further, the average diameter of axons in humans is considerably less than 0.10 mm and many are 0.001 mm. Large-diameter axons conduct information faster than small-diameter axons.

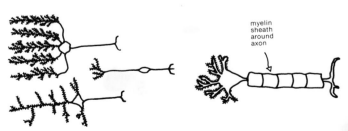

There is an enormous variety of neuron shapes and sizes.

Many neurons have a layer of myelin on their axons.

Many axons are covered with myelin, a thin layer of white insulating cells. Myelinated axons transmit information about 10 times faster than unmyelinated axons of the same diameter. Multiple sclerosis is characterized by a progressive loss of myelin, which results in slowed transmission, with consequent behavioural and physiological disturbances. Initially there is a loss of feeling, particularly in the hands and feet. Muscular weakness and partial blindness follow.

1.3 Structural organization of neurons

The dendrites of every neuron receive input from many other neurons. The axon of each neuron can terminate on many other neurons. It has been estimated that each neuron in the human nervous system receives input from about 10,000 other neurons.

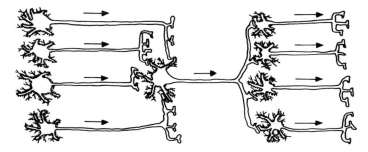

The arrows show the normal direction of information flow between neurons — from the axon of one neuron to the dendrites of the next.

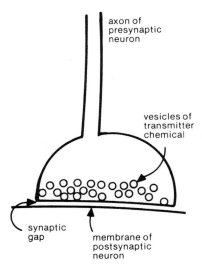

axon of presynaptic neuron

vesicles of transmitter chemical

synaptic gap

membrane of postsynaptic neuron

A close-up view of one junction, a *synapse*, between two neurons. The end of the axon contains many bundles (vesicles) of transmitter chemical.

The junction between two neurons is called a *synapse*. The axon usually widens at this junction, forming a series of small knobs called synaptic knobs or varicosities. The varicosities do not make contact anatomically with the next cell. However, the varicosities contain thousands of *vesicles* which contain chemicals. These chemicals are called *neurotransmitters*, because they convey or transmit information from one nerve cell to another.

1.4 The reception and transmission of information

Although most neurophysiological information has been collected from research with simple invertebrates such as the squid and cockroach, the general principles are similar for all species and for almost all nerve cells.

When a stimulus strikes a receptor, the energy of the stimulus is changed or *transduced* into neural energy. How this transduction occurs differs for each receptor, and in many cases is not known. Nevertheless, it is possible to look at the result of the transduction without knowing its exact mechanisms.

The fluid inside both receptors and neurons has a chemical composition different from the fluid outside the nerve cells. The fluid inside contains large, negatively charged organic ions which tend to give the cell a constant negative electrical potential. This

Information is transmitted in the nervous system by means of brief electrical impulses which are actively propagated along the axons of neurons.

The fluid inside nerve cells is chemically different from the fluid outside nerve cells. The different chemical composition results in an electrical potential difference between the inside and outside of the cell. Thus each cell is polarized.

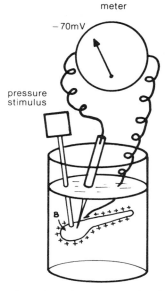

A hypothetical experiment showing
electrical potential difference between
the inside and outside of a cell.

is partially balanced by an abundance of positively charged potassium ions. In contrast, the outside has a relative abundance of
positively charged sodium ions.

The difference in ionic distribution results in a small
difference in electrical potential (voltage) between the inside and
the outside of the cell. This electrical potential difference is
called the *resting potential*. The inside of the cell is usually about
70 thousandths of a volt (70 millivolts or 70 mV) more negatively
charged than the outside of the cell. Therefore we speak of the
cell as being *polarized*. Most cells are polarized, however the
ability of various events to cause changes in the polarity of nerve
cells is unique. It is this "excitability" which underlies the
unique ability of the cells to conduct and process information.

Assume that we have isolated a pressure receptor and suspended it in fluid identical to the fluid in which it normally exists.
This would allow us to pass a fine recording electrode through
the membrane and into the cytoplasm of the cell. If the electrode
were connected to a voltmeter, it would indicate an electrical
potential difference (voltage) between the inside and outside of
the cell.

If weak pressure is applied briefly to the cell, it will cause
the resting potential of the cell to change in the direction of
becoming less negative (from, say, –70mV to –65mV). The pressure causes the membrane to become more permeable at that
point, resulting in a small depolarization. If the pressure stimulus
is removed, the membrane processes will rapidly restore the
–70 mV resting potential. A slightly stronger stimulus causes a
slightly larger change (for example, from –70 mV to –60 mV).

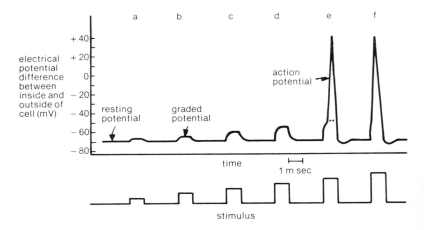

The electrical potential changes as brief and gradually increasing strength
pressure stimuli are administered to a single pressure receptor.

The small changes in the cell's resting potential reflect the strength of the stimulus in a graded manner, and they are thus called *graded potentials*. These small voltage changes are often termed *local graded potentials* since they do not spread far along the cell membrane. If the pressure probe is moved further away from the recording electrode to point B there will be no detectable change in the resting potential during the stimulation.

If, for successive stimuli, the intensity of the pressure is increased systematically, for weak stimuli the size of the graded potential increases, as in the diagram. In case *e*, the dotted line shows the expected increase if we merely extrapolate from the earlier increases. However the result obtained in *e* is quite different.

If the stimulus is strong enough to drive the potential difference between the inside and outside of the cell to -50 mV, a point called the *threshold*, a radical change in the permeability of the membrane occurs. It suddenly becomes massively permeable, and sodium ions rush into the cell. The difference in potential briefly shoots up to +40 mV and then returns to the resting level (-70 mV). This dramatic change is called an *action potential* or, because of its appearance on an oscilloscope, a *spike*. When an action potential or spike occurs, the cell is said to have *fired*.

Once the breakdown of the cell membrane permeability occurs at one point, it affects the point immediately next to it. The permeability at this point in turn breaks down and affects the next point, and so on. Thus the action potential travels from point to point along the cell membrane in the manner of a chain reaction. The size of the action potential transmitted along the axon is maintained at a constant level, since the permeability of the membrane continues to break down to exactly the same extent.

The breakdown in membrane permeability during an action potential is momentary. At each point the membrane breaks down for approximately one-thousandth of a second, after which its relatively impermeable resting state is recovered. The regeneration process is referred to as *active propagation* of the action potential.

Not all stimuli produce action potentials. When the stimulus in our example was not strong enough to cause the resting potential to exceed the threshold, only a local graded potential occurred — a small change which extinguishes in a restricted area of the membrane. A stimulus less than the threshold is referred to as *subthreshold*; one of greater than threshold intensity is called *suprathreshold*.

Action potentials (or spikes) normally move only in the direction from cell-body to axon, and active propagation ensures that the action potentials stay the same size as they move along the axon. Therefore, if a cell fires, it produces a fixed-size action potential which travels at a fixed speed. These two principles of

Weak stimuli cause small changes in the resting potential of the membrane close to the stimulus. These small changes in potential are called local graded potentials.

If the change in resting potential is large enough, then the membrane effectively 'breaks' and a massive change in potential occurs. This massive change is called an action potential or nerve impulse.

The 'break' affects the membrane next to it, which in turn 'breaks' and so on. Thus the action potential travels along the cell.

The action potential is effectively a leak, and this 'leak' travels down the axon away from the cell body.

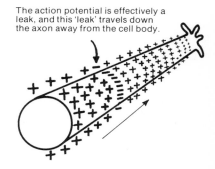

A representation of an action potential or nerve impulse travelling down the axon of a cell towards the nerve terminals.

The size and speed of the action potential or nerve impulse remains the same as it travels along the cell.

invariance of spike size and conduction speed are sometimes collectively referred to as the "all or none law". Consequently, the size of an action potential and its speed of conduction are not affected by the strength of the stimulus and thus cannot convey information about, or "code", stimulus strength.

However it is obvious that we can detect changes in stimulus strength. Therefore we must consider other means by which these changes are neurally coded. Coding principles for stimulus dimensions such as shape, colour, etc. will be considered in Chapter 5.

To study the effect of stimulus intensity on transmission, we return to the laboratory example. If we had used a stronger stimulus than *e*, say *f* in the diagram, an action potential would be generated in almost the same way as for *e*. Careful study would show that it occurred a little sooner than *e*, but this would not be obvious to casual observation. To differentiate the effects of two stimuli of different strength, it is necessary to monitor the activity of the cell over a longer period of time. It then becomes apparent that increasing the strength of the stimulus increases the *number* of spikes (or firing rate) initiated by the stimulus. Again we stress that, while a stronger stimulus increases firing rate, the size and conduction velocity of the resulting action potentials is the same for any suprathreshold stimulus.

Increasing the strength of the stimulus increases the number of action potentials in a given time.

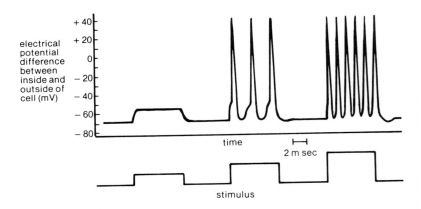

electrical potential difference between inside and outside of cell (mV)

Increasing stimulus strength increases the *number* of action potentials which occur.

Once an action potential is initiated, it takes a little time for the cell to recover its resting potential (repolarize) before another action potential can be initiated. The recovery time, or *refractory period*, limits the number of action potentials that can be initiated and travel along a neuron in a second. In other words, the refractory period limits the neuron's maximum firing rate — its maximum rate of information transfer. The highest firing rates reported have been about 1000 spikes per second.

The recovery time after an action potential is called the refractory period.

The above discussion suggests that, if the permeal ility of the membrane can be prevented from "breaking down", no action potentials will be initiated and thus no information will be transmitted by that cell. This is the mode of action of some local anaesthetics. By preventing the breakdown in the permeability of the membrane, transmission of information about painful stimuli to the central nervous system is prevented.

Local anaesthetics prevent membrane breakdown and thus block transmission of neural information.

It is tempting to think of the brain as a computer, and neural transmission as being similar to the transmission of electricity. Such an analogy is wrong. Wires are passive vehicles for the electrical signal, whereas every point along the axon of a neuron actively *regenerates* the impulse as it travels along. The difference is even more clear in terms of the relative speeds of neural and electrical conduction. Electricity travels at about 3×10^8 m/sec, whereas the fastest conduction of a nerve impulse is at least one million times slower (about 300 m/sec).

1.5 Transmission between cells

The space between two nerve cells is called the synaptic gap or synaptic cleft. This gap is extremely narrow — usually about 0.00005 mm. The synaptic cleft prevents a pre-synaptic action potential from jumping between the two cells. Instead, the action potential causes the nerve terminals to release certain chemicals which diffuse rapidly across the cleft where they can then alter the membrane permeability of the post-synaptic cell. Thus we see that transmission of information within cells is an electrical process, whereas transmission of information between cells is a chemical process. Therefore, information transmission in the nervous system is, in effect, an *electrochemical* process.

Transmission of information between cells is a chemical process. Action potentials cause the neuron to release neurotransmitter chemicals from its terminals into the synaptic gap.

Neurotransmitters are stored in pre-synaptic vesicles which prevent them from being destroyed by enzymes in the nerve

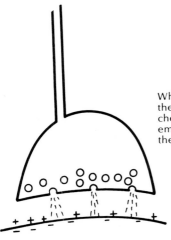

When an action potential comes down the axon, the bundles of transmitter chemical move to the membrane and empty the transmitter chemical into the synaptic gap.

terminal. This biochemical "packaging" keeps the neuro-transmitters in a state of readiness for mobilization by action potentials.

The action potentials cause the vesicles to move towards the pre-synaptic membrane. It is thought that when the vesicles contact the pre-synaptic membrane, they combine with it and empty the neurotransmitters into the synaptic cleft. The neuro-transmitters diffuse rapidly across the cleft where they then com-bine with receptors on the post-synaptic cell membrane. When a neurotransmitter occupies a receptor site, it initiates a complex sequence of events that alters the resting potential of the post-synaptic cell. Although the above example relates to commu-nication between neurons, similar processes occur during both receptor–neuron and neuron–effector communication.

The neurotransmitter chemicals change the resting potential of the next cell.

The amount of neurotransmitter released from a nerve termi-nal by one action potential produces only a small change in the resting potential of the post-synaptic cell. To drive the resting potential of that cell to its firing threshold requires the combined effects of many action potentials.

The combined effect of many action potentials is usually needed to cause an action potential in the next cell.

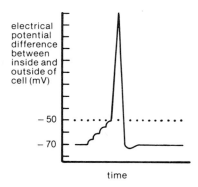

electrical potential difference between inside and outside of cell (mV)

— 50

— 70

time

Summation can drive the resting potential of the post-synaptic cell above the threshold and so trigger an action potential. Each 'step' in the graph shows the effect of an extra amount of neurotransmitter. These 'steps' can combine or summate to produce an action potential.

The summation can take place either by the simultaneous efforts of a number of different nerve terminals acting at different places on the post-synaptic cell, or by the sequential effects of a rapid volley of impulses at one nerve terminal. The two processes are respectively called *spatial summation* and *temporal summation*. Since most cells probably fire as the result of both processes, one could view neuronal firing as reflecting spatiotemporal summation.

The processes described above tend to depict neurons as being generally inactive in the absence of appropriate stimulation.

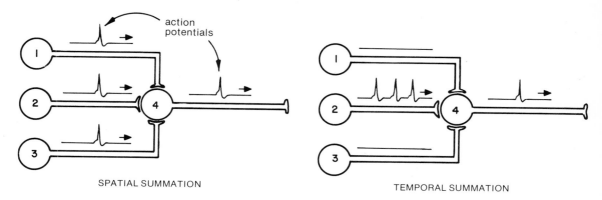

SPATIAL SUMMATION   TEMPORAL SUMMATION

Spatial summation (left). If action potentials from cells 1, 2 and 3 arrive at cell 4 simultaneously, then they may release sufficient transmitter to trigger an action potential in cell 4. Temporal summation (right). If action potentials from one cell arrive in rapid succession then sufficient transmitter may be released to trigger an action potential in the next cell (the post-synaptic cell). Either type of summation can drive the resting potential of the post-synaptic cell above the threshold and so trigger an action potential in it.

However, most nerve cells are spontaneously active and maintain a certain firing rate even when all inputs are removed. Inputs simply change the background firing rate of the post-synaptic cell.

Spontaneous activity refers to the occurrence of action potentials in the absence of any input.

Neurotransmitters do not always decrease the resting potential of the post-synaptic cell. In some cases they increase its resting potential making it more negative and thus less likely to fire. In such a case we could say that the neurotransmitter has had an inhibitory effect. Rather than a particular neurotransmitter always being excitatory or inhibitory, it appears that the net effect (excitation or inhibition) of any neurotransmitter is determined by the nature of that transmitter, and also by the characteristics of the post-synaptic receptors.

Some transmitter chemicals make the resting potential of the next cell more negative. These are called inhibitory transmitters since they tend to prevent or inhibit nerve impulses.

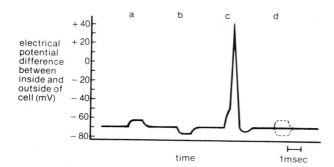

Some neurotransmitters *decrease* the negative resting potential of the post-synaptic cell (a). They are said to have an excitatory effect. Other neurotransmitters *increase* the negative resting potential of the post-synaptic cell (b). They are said to have an inhibitory effect and can cancel the excitatory effects of other neurotransmitters (d).

Each neuron can receive a variety of transmitter chemicals.

Most nerve cells seem to contain only the one transmitter chemical, although recently there have been some reports of nerve cells which apparently contain two or more. However, each nerve cell can *receive* a variety of transmitter chemicals. Apparently, all over the membrane of the nerve cell there are receptor sites specialized to receive different kinds of transmitter chemical. Whether any one cell transmits an action potential depends on the relative effects from all these receptors on the cell membrane.

In summary, nerve cells are often spontaneously active and this activity is modulated (increased or decreased) by inputs from other cells. Whether the modulation is in the direction of *excitation* (increased firing rate) or *inhibition* (decreased firing rate) is dependent upon the sum of excitatory and inhibitory inputs.

1.6 Transmission at the neuromuscular junction

At the end of each neural network, information passes from a neuron to an effector cell. Just as there is a gap between other links in the nervous system, so there is a gap between the axon of the last neuron and the muscle cell. This is the neuromuscular junction. When an action potential comes down the axon, a transmitter (acetylcholine) is released into the neuromuscular junction and the neurotransmitter causes the contraction of the muscle cell. Muscles consist of many individual cells, and an observable muscular response arises from the simultaneous contraction of a large number of muscle cells. Sustained muscular contraction requires a continuous stream of activation, and thus chemical action at the junction is of critical importance.

The junction between the axon of a neuron and muscle cell is called a neuromuscular junction.

1.7 The metabolism of neurotransmitters

Drugs which alter neurotransmitter activity may affect behaviour, perception and thinking.

Every sensation, perception or thought, and every physiological or behavioural response depends on microchemical events. Dramatic changes in perception and behaviour resulting from the modulation, by drugs, of neurotransmitter activity is one of the most powerful, exciting and potentially dangerous discoveries man has ever made. A key to understanding this rapidly expanding area, *psychopharmacology*, lies in the understanding of the life cycle or metabolism of neurotransmitters.

Neurotransmitter metabolism can be discussed under three main headings: (1) synthesis; (2) storage and release; and (3) inactivation. Storage and release have been discussed in section 1.5, and as synthesis and inactivation will be discussed in detail in later chapters, we shall at present consider only the more general principles.

A list of suspected neurotransmitters indicating the general chemical groups to which they belong, their most common names and abbreviations. This list is necessarily incomplete since some of the more disputed candidates such as the prostaglandins, histamine and the cyclic nucleotides have been omitted. Further, it is likely that many more amino acid and peptide transmitters will be discovered in the near future.

CHEMICAL CLASS	NEUROTRANSMITTER NAME
Quaternary Amine	acetylcholine (Ach)
Catecholamines	dopamine (DA)
	noradrenalin (NA)*
	adrenalin (A)**
Indoleamines	serotonin (5-HT)***
	melatonin
Amino Acids	gamma aminobutyric acid (GABA)
	glycine
	glutamic acid
Peptides	substance P
	enkephalins
	endorphins

*   usually called norepinephrine (NE) in the U.S.A.
**   usually called epinephrine (E) in the U.S.A.
***   the abbreviation 5-HT is derived from the proper chemical name 5-hydroxytryptamine

Most presently suspected neurotransmitters are either amino acids or are synthesized from amino acids. Although some amino acids may be synthesized in the brain, it appears that the majority are obtained from the breakdown of food proteins. Thus dietary factors can potentially influence behaviour by regulating the availability of these precursors of neurotransmitters. However, this should not be misinterpreted as supporting "brain diets" or "psychodietetics". Under most conditions, precursor availability is a relatively minor factor in the regulation of neurotransmitter metabolism.

Amino acids are the 'building blocks' of neurotransmitters.

Amino acids are transported by the blood stream from the gastro-intestinal tract to the brain where they are extracted by energy-dependent uptake mechanisms. Once inside the neurons, the amino acids undergo a series of chemical reactions, each requiring certain enzymes, which convert them into neuro-transmitters. Presumably, the amino acid transmitters are packaged into vesicles and transported to the nerve terminals. At the moment little is known about the metabolism of either the amino acid transmitters or the more recently discovered *peptide* transmitters.

Once released into the synaptic cleft, the action of the various neurotransmitters is rapidly terminated by chemical and physiological means. Chemical termination is achieved by enzymes which transform the neurotransmitters into inactive (or at least less active) products called *metabolites*. The metabolites may in turn be broken down and eventually excreted from the

Once released into the synapse, neuro-transmitter chemicals act on the next cell and are then broken down by enzymes or taken back into the original cell ('re-uptake').

Measuring neurotransmitter residues in body fluids gives a guide to neurotransmitter operation.

body. Consequently, measuring the levels of selected transmitter metabolites in the blood, cerebrospinal fluid, urine, saliva and so on provides an index of the activity of a particular transmitter system in the brain. Because of the ease with which blood and urine samples can be taken, the analysis of metabolites in these fluids is a widely used clinical and experimental index of brain function. However this is an indirect measure and may be confounded by many extraneous variables.

Physiological termination of neurotransmitter action involves the re-uptake of the transmitter into the pre-synaptic terminal. It may be thought of as a neurochemical recycling process, in which the unmetabolized transmitter is "repackaged" and released again.

The relative importance of enzymatic versus re-uptake inactivation varies according to the particular neurotransmitter system. For example, acetylcholine is inactivated by an enzyme (acetylcholinesterase), whereas noradrenalin is primarily inactivated by re-uptake. The enzymes monoamine oxidase (MAO) and catechol-o-methyl transferase serve a relatively minor role in the inactivation of noradrenalin.

If either of these inactivation mechanisms malfunctions, serious disturbances in neural and, consequently, physiological and behavioural processes can occur. For example, the inactivation of the enzyme acetylcholinesterase at the neuromuscular junction results in a surplus of acetylcholine and the overactivation of the muscle. It is in this manner that nerve gases and snake venoms exert their toxic effects. By preventing transmitter breakdown, they cause sustained muscle activation which manifests itself as violent and uncontrollable muscle spasms that may result in death. Insecticides of the organophosphate variety block transmitter breakdown in insect nervous systems and, in high doses, are similarly toxic in humans.

The disease myasthenia gravis involves defective transmission at the neuromuscular junction. People suffering from the disease cannot activate their muscles for any prolonged effort. They start a handshake firmly but cannot maintain the effort and the hand quickly goes limp.

In later chapters we shall see that a variety of abnormalities in transmitter metabolism have been associated with phenomena as diverse as migraine headaches and schizophrenia. By understanding the metabolic disturbances, we may then be able to use drugs which will either eliminate the disturbances, or at least compensate for them. In the past decade, pharmacological developments resulting from basic neurochemical research have provided dramatic therapeutic advances.

Questions

1 What are the names given to the major parts of a neuron?
2 What is myelin and what is its function?
3 Why is the membrane of nerve cells so important?
4 What is meant by resting potential, graded potentials, action potentials?
5 How does a nerve impulse travel along a cell?
6 Why is −50 mV important in relation to a nerve impulse?
7 What is the "all-or-none" law?
8 How does stimulus strength affect neural response?
9 What is the refractory period?
10 How is information transmitted from one cell to another?
11 What are spatial and temporal summation?
12 What is spontaneous activity?
13 What happens to neurotransmitters once they have been released?

Further Readings

Cotman, C.W. and McGaugh, J.L. *Behavioral Neuroscience*. New York, Academic Press. 1980
Cowan, W.M. The development of the brain. *Scientific American*, 1979. **241** (3), 106–117.
Iversen, L.L. The chemistry of the brain. *Scientific American*, 1979, **241** (3), 118–129.
Katz, B. *Nerve, Muscle and Synapse*. New York, McGraw-Hill, 1966.
Kuffler, S.W. and Nicolls, J.G. *From Neuron to Brain — A Cellular Approach to the Function of the Nervous System*.
    Sunderland, Mass., Sinauer. 1976.

2

Research Techniques in Neuroscience

2.1 Introduction

The brain could be thought of as an homogenous mass of neurons, with neurons concerned with particular functions uniformly spread throughout it. Fortunately this is not the case. Cells serving a particular function tend to be grouped together. For example, all the cell bodies of the neurons which synapse on and directly control the muscle cells of the lateral muscle in the right eye are grouped together in a 1 mm^3 region in the right half of the brain stem, called the abducens nucleus. The location of this nucleus is similar in all human beings. In turn, the neurons of the abducens nucleus receive information from other groups of cells throughout the brain.

Neurons serving particular functions tend to be grouped together.

Since neurons tend to be grouped together in nuclei it has made study of the brain considerably easier than it otherwise might have been. Knowing where these cell-bodies are and where their axons project has meant that it is possible to start making "wiring diagrams" of the brain. For example, it has been possible to verify the function of the neurons of the abducens nucleus by electrically stimulating them through fine electrodes and observing the resulting eye movement. Further verification has come from implanting even finer microelectrodes into the nucleus and recording the action potentials in single abducens neurons during eye movements.

Some neuroscientists endeavour to make 'wiring diagrams' of parts of the brain.

But from where do the neurons of the abducens nucleus receive *their* input to make the eyes move? Clearly we have to move further back along the neural chain. But how? One way is to use neuroanatomical methods. For example, tracer chemicals injected in the region of a nucleus can be taken up by the axons which terminate there and transported back along these axons where they concentrate in the cell-bodies of these earlier neurons. One such tracer is called horseradish peroxidase. Appropriate treatment makes cell-bodies containing this enzyme stain differently compared to cell-bodies without it.

The information gained by this means can be confirmed by other techniques using radioactive isotopes injected around the earlier cell-bodies. These isotopes are transported *down* the axons and are concentrated at the axon terminals. Again appropriate treatment shows where the axons of the injected cell-bodies terminate. This technique is called *autoradiography*.

Neuroanatomical methods only tell us *where* groups of cells are. They tell us nothing about the information these cells convey. To find out the *functions* of nerve cells one needs information from recording and electrical stimulation studies.

Neuroanatomical techniques give information about location, not function.

In turn one can ask from where do these earlier cells receive *their* information and what exactly is this information. To answer these questions we have to apply anatomical tracing, stimulating and recording techniques all over again, further back in the system.

In contrast to these systematic tracing techniques stand other methods which seek more general answers to questions about widespread activity patterns throughout the brain. For example, a very recent technique using radioactively labelled glucose has allowed investigators to see which parts of the brain have been active. The labelled glucose accumulates in active cells, and after appropriate treatment the regions which have been active literally light up. This is called the 2-deoxyglucose technique.

The use of radioactively tagged glucose now allows visualization of areas of the brain that are active.

An entirely different approach has been to treat the brain so that all neurons containing a particular chemical transmitter are made to fluoresce. Again, however, the *functions* of these fluorescent cells are not established by such a procedure, but it does show widespread systems of neurochemically defined pathways.

Fluorescence techniques show the location of certain neurotransmitters.

A basic limitation of all the above neuroanatomical procedures is that they require removal of the brain. Consequently such techniques have only very limited applicability in the study of the human brain. Recent developments in nuclear medicine and computers have provided two new and exciting methods of non-invasively investigating the human brain.

Computer assisted tomography (CAT), which is more commonly known as a brain scan, is an application of X-ray techniques. By serially scanning the brain in two planes at right angles to each other this technique feeds information to a computer which constructs a three dimensional representation of the brain. This technique is sufficiently powerful to show local changes in blood flow, presumably reflecting changes in neuronal activity, in association with a variety of human behaviours. Similarly, CAT frequently permits quite precise delineation of areas of brain damage produced by tumours or strokes.

There is another technique related to CAT which may eventually be much more useful. *Positron emission tomography* (PET) is a scanning technique based on positron emitting isotopes of any of a variety of elements of the brain. With PET it is, in theory, possible to follow the activity of a single neurotransmitter anywhere in a living human brain. The main drawback with PET at the moment is its enormous expense. Since the positron emitting isotopes have extremely short life-spans, it is necessary to have an on-site cyclotron to make the isotopes. Also, the scanning equipment and computer cost millions of dollars. For these reasons PET will remain a generally unavailable, though highly desirable, technique for some time.

2.2 Histological techniques

After the experiment the site of the stimulating or recording electrode must be identified. This procedure is called histological verification.

Functional information must be complemented by anatomical information. For example, when an experiment is completed we must verify that the electrode was really in the intended nucleus. There is a wide variety of methods we can use for precisely verifying electrode locations as well as for describing the structure and interconnections by various brain areas. Collectively they are referred to as *histological* techniques.

Histological techniques require that the brain be removed and treated so that it can be cut in very thin slices before treating these slices to highlight various cellular details. The brain is often treated with a fixative (such as formalin or alcohol) to prevent deterioration. Then, it must be hardened, usually by freezing or embedding it in paraffin or plastic, to permit thin sections (typically 1–40 μm) to be taken (1 μm = 0.001 mm). The sectioning is done on a slicing device called a *microtome*.

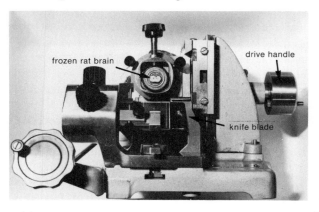

frozen rat brain

drive handle

knife blade

A typical freezing microtome with a piece of rat brain mounted on its moveable stage. Operating the drive handle on the right brings the tissue into contact with the blade, thus cutting a thin section.

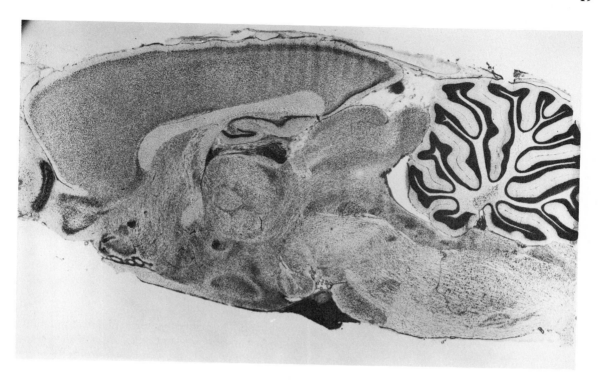

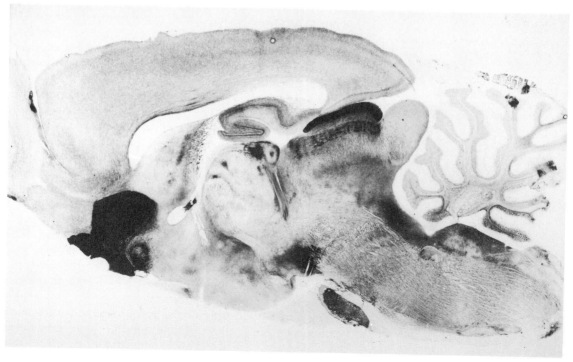

Parasagittal sections of rat brain with section (A) stained to highlight cell bodies and section (B) stained to highlight fibre tracts. The rat's snout would be on the left.

Finally, the section may be processed by any one of many hundreds of techniques to enable the visualization of cellular details and interconnections. Without such treatment brain tissue has remarkably few visible distinguishing features.

In order to highlight the various features in which we may be interested, different stains are used. For example, certain dyes, such as toluidine blue-O, stain the neuron cell-body. Brain tissue stained with such dyes reveals numerous clusters of cell-bodies. A distinct cluster of cell-bodies is called a nucleus. (Try not to confuse this with the nucleus that each individual cell has.) Other dyes, such as oil red-O, stain the myelin sheath that covers many axons. Tissue stained with such dyes reveals groups of axons. Often these groups of axons follow a similar course. Such groups of axons are called fibre tracts. Nuclei and fibre tracts are the major elements of traditional neuroanatomy.

2.3 Stereotaxic surgery

A basic problem in applying direct experimental manipulation to the brain is that we can only see superficial areas of the cerebral cortex. The great mass of the brain is hidden beneath the cortex. To expose these subcortical areas it would be necessary to remove all of the brain tissue above. If this were done the effects of any experimental manipulation to a subcortical area would be obscured by the damage required to expose it. Stereotaxic surgery was developed to allow the positioning of probes (electrodes or cannulae) in subcortical areas while only inflicting minimal damage to overlying tissue.

Stereotaxic surgery makes use of a stereotaxic instrument and a three-dimensional set of coordinates which specifies the location of any site in the brain in relation to certain reference points. The coordinates are obtained from a brain atlas which is a set of calibrated slices through the brain.

There are many types of stereotaxic instruments, and these have certain features in common. One is the *head holder*, which is used to fix the skull in a standard position corresponding to the plane of orientation of the brain atlas being used. The head holder typically consists of rigidly mounted tapered bars, which are inserted into the external ear holes, and a bite bar, which holds the snout in place. With the head thus secured the location of any site in the brain may be specified in relation to reference points on the stereotaxic instrument.

The actual positioning of the probe is done with a micromanipulator which allows precise movements in three dimensions. Basically, a small entry hole is made in the rigidly mounted skull and the micromanipulator is then used to insert the probe to the desired subcortical location. This technique allows access

Stereotaxic procedures permit study of structures deep in the brain, with minimal damage to the surface layers of the brain.

Stereotaxic instruments use three-dimensional geometry to guide a probe deep into the brain.

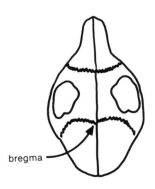

bregma

Looking down on a guinea pig skull. The joins between the bones make fine lines and one junction is used as a reference point (bregma).

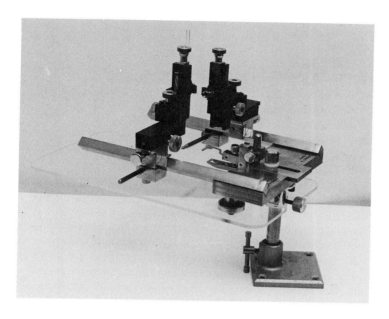

A stereotaxic instrument which is used for holding an animal's head in a known, repeatable position.

to any subcortical area, yet it entails only minimal damage to overlying brain tissue. The extent of this entry damage is determined by the size of the probe.

While stereotaxic instruments for human brain surgery are essentially similar to that described above, the determination of stereotaxic coordinates for human surgery is quite different. Stereotaxic atlases for laboratory species depend upon various brain structures bearing a constant spatial relationship to the skull. Since laboratory species are carefully selected for their structural homogeneity, the atlases are quite accurate for these species. However, in working with humans the surgeon is faced with large individual differences in skull–brain relationships. To circumvent this problem, human stereotaxic coordinates are individually determined by X-ray and electrophysiological techniques.

2.4 Techniques for inactivating parts of the brain

The simplest way to inactivate a part of the brain is to remove it. Neurosurgeons often have to remove parts of the brain from patients with brain tumours or epilepsy. Similarly, disease, accidents and bullets can all cause brain damage. Much has been learned about brain function by relating changes in behaviour to the region and extent of brain damage. But with human patients

Ablation is removal of brain matter. The term lesion refers to a damaged part of the brain.

An electrode is a probe used to conduct electricity. Passing direct current through an electrode into the brain can cause a lesion.

Temporary inactivation of neural tissue can be achieved by localized cooling.

Some toxins selectively destroy neurons containing a particular transmitter.

it is rare to have precise information about the person's behaviour before the brain damage, and often there is little precise information about the location and extent of the lesion. Because of such problems, the effects of lesions may be examined more systematically in laboratory animals.

The technique for removal of part of the brain is called *ablation* or *extirpation*. One way to do this is by *suction*. This technique requires visual guidance and, unless radiographic techniques are used, it is virtually impossible to remove subcortical regions by suction without causing extensive damage to overlying cortical regions of the brain.

Brain tissue can also be inactivated by electrical means. To do this, an electrode is inserted into the brain so that its tip is in the region to be inactivated. An electrode is any probe that is used to conduct electricity. It is usually a piece of wire covered with insulation, except at its tip. Most electrodes are small in diameter so that damage to overlying brain structures is generally minimized. If direct current is passed through the electrode, electrolysis occurs at the tip, destroying nearby brain cells and creating an *electrolytic lesion*. If an alternating high-frequency current is passed through the electrode, heat is produced around the tip, destroying neighbouring cells and creating a *radiofrequency lesion*. Both techniques produce roughly spherical areas of damage, their size being determined largely by the size of the electrode tip and the strength and duration of the current. Other techniques for producing lesions are focused gamma rays and ultrasonic vibration. Nerve cells in the region of the focus are destroyed, leaving nerve cells in overlying structures relatively undamaged.

In contrast with these irreversible lesion techniques, it is often desirable to make reversible lesions. Such techniques make a particular brain area functionally inoperative for a short time with no permanent effects. This can be done by cooling or by injection of a local anaesthetic directly into the brain area under investigation.

Just as there are histological techniques to visualize certain neurotransmitters, there are also lesion techniques that produce a relatively selective destruction of neurons containing a particular transmitter. An example of such a specific neurotoxin is 6-hydroxydopamine (6-OHDA). 6-OHDA injected into the brain is picked up almost exclusively by dopaminergic neurons. Once inside the neuron this toxin interferes with normal metabolic processes and destroys the neuron. This technique permits an examination of the functional role of dopaminergic neurons that is relatively uncomplicated by destruction of other neurons. There are other neurotoxic procedures that are relatively specific to noradrenergic and serotonergic neurons. Experimental use of these neurotoxins has generated a great deal of valuable data on the role of the biogenic amines in a variety of behavioural and physiological processes.

There are, however, a number of non-selective neurotoxins that unfortunately produce their destructive effects even when taken orally. Examples of these are the heavy metals, lead, mercury and cadmium. These substances sometimes enter the food chain through industrial "accidents", although often their dumping is quite intentional. For example, a great deal of the high levels of lead that appear in many foodstuffs originates from ethyl lead which is a widely used petroleum additive.

The heavy metals are neurochemically blind in that they will destroy any neuron that picks them up. Unlike many other forms of tissue damage neurotoxic destruction is permanent and irreversible. Until adequate environmental safeguards are implemented, we will continue to inflict unnecessary brain damage on many thousands of people annually.

For lesions caused by either ablation, electrical or neurotoxic means, histological verification of the location and extent of the lesion is necessary. Apart from technical problems such as scar formation or tissue infection, the interpretation of lesion results is difficult. A lesion may cause changed behaviour, depending on its site, for a number of reasons. For example, it may cause a sensory loss, or motor difficulties, or affect the animal's attention, its memory, or its appetite. In order to decide which of the possibilites is correct, it is usually necessary to examine the behaviour carefully and to run additional tests and control conditions.

Brain lesions can alter behaviour for a variety of reasons. Careful observation and experiment are needed to understand the effect of the lesion.

2.5 Techniques for activating parts of the brain

Electrical stimulation. An electrode is stereotaxically inserted into the brain region to be studied. The electrode is fixed to a socket which is attached rigidly to the skull. After the animal has recovered, we can study the effect of electrical stimulation by plugging leads into the socket and giving the animal weak electrical stimulation. The electrical stimulation passes through the socket, down the electrode and affects neurons around the uninsulated tip of the electrode. If a small current alternating at low frequency is passed through the electrode, no lesion is formed, but the electrical activity of neurons around the tip of the electrode may be increased.

Passing weak alternating current through an electrode into the brain activates neurons around the tip of the electrode.

Electrical stimulation of the brain has been used extensively in studies on animals, but it has also been used on humans, for example with patients undergoing surgical treatment for severe epilepsy. Epilepsy is apparently caused by regions of abnormal brain activity. Should such abnormal activity spread to other regions of the brain, an epileptic seizure may result. During a major seizure the patient loses consciousness and the body

Epilepsy is caused by regions of abnormal brain activity.

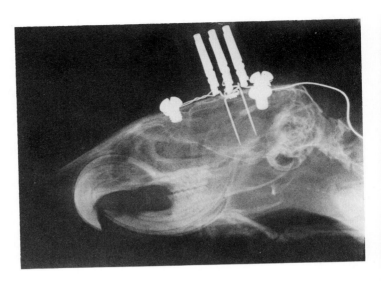

An X-ray of electrodes implanted into a rat's brain.

One treatment of extremely severe epilepsy is to remove the abnormal brain tissue.

stiffens, and then there is a rhythmic shaking of the limbs and body. This whole sequence is usually completed in a minute or two after which the patient is confused and drowsy. Anti-epileptic drugs generally prevent the spreading of the abnormal neural activity. However, some severe epilepsies do not respond satisfactorily to drug therapy. In these cases the epilepsy may be alleviated by surgical removal of the abnormal brain tissue.

During these operations, which were pioneered by Penfield and Rasmussen, the surgeon uses electrical stimulation of the brain surface to discover which parts of the brain are suspect and which regions should be spared if possible. Under general anaesthesia a large flap of bone is removed, exposing the cortex. The patient is then allowed to regain consciousness, and pain is prevented by injection of local anaesthetic around the incision. An electrode is placed on the cortex and a small burst of current is used to excite the neurons around the tip of the electrode. The characteristics of the brain stimulation are carefully selected so that the stimulation does not damage the brain tissue. Being conscious, the patient can report the sensations produced by electrical stimulation. The surgeon is thus able to observe the responses elicited by the stimulation of different sites in order to detect the site which, when lesioned, is likely to give the patient optimum relief. The stimulation is not painful since there are no pain receptors in the cortex.

Electrical stimulation of specific areas of the cortex causes limb movements or sensations of being touched.

Electrical stimulation of the brain has also been used with a few blind patients. This research has shown that they can perceive visual sensations when brief current pulses are applied to electrodes in contact with the visual area of the brain. One particular train of pulses delivered to an electrode results in the perception of a spot of light, called a phosphene, in a particular location in space. The higher the current, the brighter the phosphene appears. A few dozen phosphenes produced by appropriately located electrodes can present simple visual patterns.

Chemical stimulation. In place of an electrode, a thin tube called a *cannula* can be inserted stereotaxically into the brain and fixed to the skull. After the animal has recovered from the insertion of the cannula, minute quantities of chemicals can then be applied. These chemicals can selectively affect neurons around the tip of the cannula. Some chemicals increase the activity of neurons, whereas others decrease it.

A cannula is a thin tube for applying chemicals directly into the brain.

Although histological examination can verify the location of the electrode or cannula, it is difficult to know which neurons have had their activity altered. Thus one of the main interpretational difficulties with these techniques is determining the extent of the spread of the electrical or chemical stimulation.

2.6 Techniques for recording the electrical activity of neurons

When an action potential passes along a neuron, it causes a small voltage change in the immediate vicinity of that neuron. An electrode with a fine tip placed near the neuron can detect the voltage changes, which then must be amplified in order to be displayed on an oscilloscope or heard on a loudspeaker.

Single neurons are often only 5–10 μm in diameter. Therefore, to record activity of single neurons, electrodes with very fine tips (about 1–3 μm) are used. These microelectrodes can be made by etching steel pins or more easily by heating a thin glass tube and stretching it mechanically to produce a very fine pointed tip. The hole in the tip of the microelectrodes can be as small as 0.1 μm. To conduct electricity, the glass microelectrode is filled with a conducting fluid.

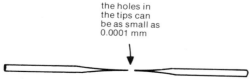

the holes in the tips can be as small as 0.0001 mm

A glass tube heated at one point and pulled apart becomes two microelectrodes, after each is filled with conducting fluid.

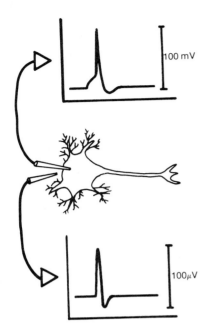

The size of action potentials picked up by a microelectrode just outside the membrane of a cell is about one thousand times smaller than if the tip is actually inside the cell.

Microelectrodes, if pushed slowly into the brain, may come sufficiently close to a neuron to detect its action potentials. The electrical activity associated with each action potential is only brief (a few thousandths of a second); hence on an oscilloscope it looks like a spike and on a loudspeaker sounds like a click. In accordance with the "all-or-none" principle, each action potential is the same size, and thus spikes from one cell are of uniform size. In this way one can determine whether the recording is from only one neuron.

By studying which stimuli affect a neuron's firing rate and how this is achieved, it is possible to determine how information is "coded" by neurons and transmitted to or from the brain (see Chapter 5).

The technical problems in single unit recording are considerable. Recording from one neuron over a period long enough to study its responses to a variety of stimuli is a formidable task. Further, histological verification of the location of the neuron, while important, can also be difficult.

Much information about single neurons has been derived from research with anaesthetized animals. However, anaesthetics affect neural activity, which can lead to misinterpretations of patterns of neural response. This problem has recently been solved in part by the use of apparently painless techniques that allow recording from single neurons in awake animals. However, these techniques are more difficult to use than recording from anaesthetized animals and are still in their infancy.

Gross electrodes have relatively large tips which can detect the activity of many neurons simultaneously. These electrodes are usually the same size as stimulating electrodes but, rather than passing current through them into the brain, the experimenter

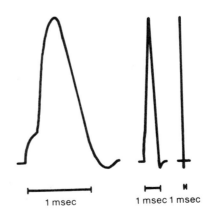

The same event — an action potential — may appear to be different because of different time scales. In this book a spike is usually used to represent an action potential.

uses the electrode to detect the continual voltage changes in the brain. If many neurons can be made to fire simultaneously by, for example, a fairly sudden stimulus, then a large "slow" response called an *evoked potential* is observed. The size of an evoked potential varies according to the number of neurons simultaneously activated. The activation of only one or two neurons would not give rise to a wave large enough to be observed.

An evoked potential is a fairly 'slow' change in neural activity picked up by large electrodes in the brain or on the scalp. It is caused by the simultaneous activation of many neurons.

Disc electrodes placed on the surface of the scalp can be used to record "brain waves" – electroencephalograph (EEG) waves. These are spontaneous rhythmic fluctuations of voltage in parts of the brain. Although widely used to diagnose abnormal brain function in both neurological and psychiatric contexts, the precise cause of the EEG remains unexplained.

The term EEG refers to weak voltages from the brain. The EEG is usually detected by disc electrodes on the scalp.

Just as the gross electrical activity of the brain can be detected by surface electrodes, the gross electrical activity of many other cell groups can be similarly recorded. For example, the electrical activity of any muscle is called the electromyogram or EMG. The electrocardiogram (ECG) and electrooculogram (EOG) are simply recordings of the electrical activity of the heart and eye respectively. When a number of these variables are recorded simultaneously they are referred to as a polygraphic recording.

2.7 Techniques for recording biological chemical activity

The activity of any nervous tissue is reflected in changes in electrical and also chemical activity. Whereas electrical stimulation and recording were discussed in sections 2.5 and 2.6, the present section is concerned with the measurement and interpretation of biochemical events. We will see that both the measurement and interpretation issues are vastly more complicated than is generally appreciated.

The activity of the brain can be studied by measuring neurochemicals (such as neurotransmitters) in parts of the brain.

The most straightforward method of determining the chemical state of the brain is to remove the brain and measure the amount of the chemicals of interest. Besides the obvious fact that this technique necessitates killing the subject, it presents other serious difficulties. Very often a behaviourally relevant neurochemical change may occur in only a small area of the brain. Whole-brain assays inevitably obscure important regional differences. The use of smaller pieces of brain tissue may circumvent this problem, but small samples require extremely sensitive analytic techniques and they also raise the problem that the experimenter may well miss the relevant area.

Another weakness of this sort of quantitative neurochemistry is that it typically uses levels of a neurotransmitter as an index of functional activity. For example, the presence of large amounts

The absolute levels of a neuro-transmitter may be a poor index of functional activity. An important determinant of functional activity is the sensitivity of the receptors for that neurotransmitter.

Measuring the breakdown products of neurochemicals in the cerebrospinal fluid (CSF) provides only a very rough guide to activity in the brain.

of the transmitter chemical dopamine in a sample is usually taken to indicate a high level of dopaminergic activity. However, recent research has shown that alterations in *receptor sensitivity* may be a more important determinant of functional activity than the amount of neurotransmitter present. Supersensitive receptors can compensate for inadequate transmitter availability, whereas subsensitive receptors can compensate for excess transmitter availability.

Methods for quantifying receptor numbers and sensitivity are still in their infancy. Some are based on the fact that the translation of information at a receptor into a change in membrane ionic permeability often involves what is known as a second messenger, an example of which is cyclic adenosine monophosphate (cAMP). Once again we arrive at the conclusion that a full appreciation of neural events is only provided by the use of a number of techniques.

Like most neuroscience research methods, brain assays are highly invasive and generally unsuitable for human studies or even for animal studies where repeated measures are required. These limitations have led to the development of a number of minimally invasive procedures which provide an indirect measure of the chemical activity of the brain.

Circulating through the central core of the brain and spinal cord is the cerebrospinal fluid (CSF). The breakdown products (metabolites) of many neurochemicals appear in the CSF, and they may be measured by puncturing the membranes around the spinal cord with a hypodermic syringe and withdrawing a sample of the CSF. However, the lumbar puncture procedure is too stressful to be routinely used in human experimentation. In addition, we only know the metabolites of a few neurotransmitters and, as discussed above, they often provide a very unclear picture of what is going on in the brain.

Essentially, similar analytic procedures can be applied to blood or urine. However, these analyses can be influenced by chemical events occurring in peripheral organs outside the nervous system. For example, metabolites of the neurotransmitter serotonin are readily detected in the blood. However, over 99% of the body's serotonin is located in the intestinal walls, where it appears to participate in intestinal motility. For this reason blood-borne serotonin metabolites tell us very little about serotonergic activity in the brain.

The case with central noradrenergic activity is more encouraging. Although there is a great deal of peripheral noradrenalin, it appears to be metabolized in a manner different from that of brain noradrenalin. The existence of the metabolite 3-methoxy-4-hydroxyphenylglycol (MHPG) in the urine may be a useful index of central noradrenalin activity.

The blood and urine are very useful for measuring hormonal activity. Small samples can be repeatedly taken and subjected to an array of exquisitely sensitive assay techniques. Such techniques have opened up new horizons of research into endocrine–behavioural interactions.

2.8 Summary

Stereotaxic techniques are a principal means of investigating the physiological basis of behaviour. These techniques enable the more precise location of cortical and subcortical regions from which recordings are to be made, or which are to be chemically or electrically stimulated, or lesioned. While the various stereotaxic techniques have been discussed in isolation, they are often used in combination with one another; for example, recording neural activity in some part of the brain in response to electrical stimulation of some other area of the brain.

After stereotaxic manipulation, brain tissue must be directly or radiographically examined to determine such factors as electrode or cannula location, and lesion size. Such histological verification enables more accurate interpretation of observed relationships between the brain and behaviour. This is essential because of the variability of brain structures within apparently homogeneous groups of subjects. Brain atlases are designed for specific strains of animals, by both age and sex. However, within groups of experimental animals there are individual differences. Thus brain atlases permit only approximate accuracy. Complementing these physiological and anatomical techniques is a wide variety of biochemical and pharmacological techniques.

Information about the function of the brain has come from many disciplines — neuroanatomy, neurophysiology, neurology, and psychology, to name a few. Each discipline has its own techniques, although clearly there is considerable overlap.

We wish to stress that every technique has its problems. There is no one "ideal" technique for studying the functions of the brain. Some techniques have more problems than others. Sometimes the problems can only be appreciated by experts, whereas in other cases the problems are widely known. Partly for this reason, the attitude we have tried to maintain in our writing and encourage in your reading is one of healthy scepticism.

There is no one 'ideal' technique for studying the functions of the brain.

There is a tendency to attach more weight to studies where the results of different techniques complement each other; for example, where neuroanatomical studies of an area are borne out by electrophysiological results on the same area, and these results are consistent with results from behavioural studies of the effects of lesioning or electrical stimulation of that area.

Questions

1   What is a group of cell-bodies called?
2   How can neural pathways be traced, and how can their function be identified?
3   How can access be obtained reliably to deep structures in the brain?
4   What is removal of part of the brain called?
5   What is a lesion?
6   How can brain lesions be made?
7   What is an electrode?
8   What effect occurs if direct current is passed into the brain?
9   What effect occurs if weak alternating current is passed into the brain?
10   How has electrical stimulation of the human brain been used clinically?

Further Readings

Myers, R.D. (Ed.) *Methods in Psychobiology* (2 vols). New York, Academic Press. 1971.
Singh, D. and Avery, D.D. *Physiological Techniques in Behavioral Research.* Monterey, Ca., Brooks–Cole. 1975.
Waynforth, H.B. *Experimental and Surgical Technique in the Rat.* London, Academic Press, 1980.

3

Neuroanatomy

3.1 The main divisions of the nervous system

The human nervous system is too complex to be discussed as a unitary system. It is therefore necessary to divide it into various subdivisions.

The main divisions of the nervous system are the *central nervous system* and the *peripheral nervous system*. The central

The central nervous system consists of the spinal cord and the brain. The remaining nervous tissue constitutes the peripheral nervous system.

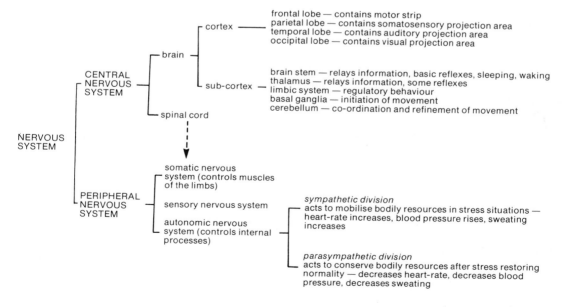

A simple classification of the divisions of the nervous system.

nervous system consists of the *spinal cord* and the *brain*. The peripheral nervous system consists of all those receptors, and afferent (input) and efferent (output) neurons whose cell-bodies lie outside the spinal cord and brain.

3.2 The peripheral nervous system

Afferent neurons convey information to the brain. Efferent neurons convey information from the brain.

The peripheral nervous system performs two main functions: it transmits information from the receptors to the central nervous system, via the *afferent* neurons, and it transmits information from the central nervous system to the effectors, via the *efferent* neurons, to enable muscular and glandular responses.

The peripheral nervous system is essentially a communication network transmitting electrochemical messages from one part of the organism to another. The difference between afferent and efferent neurons is the direction of information transfer.

The somatic nerves control skeletal muscles.

Internal organs are controlled by the autonomic nervous system.

The peripheral nervous system is further divided into *somatic* (or voluntary) and *autonomic* (self-governing or involuntary) components. The somatic (voluntary) nerves are primarily concerned with the control of skeletal muscles, which produce body movements. The autonomic (involuntary) nerves are primarily involved in the control of the muscles of internal organs such as the gut, blood vessels, heart and certain glands such as the tear glands and salivary glands. The word "autonomic" means "not under voluntary control". Recently, however, by giving subjects feedback about their autonomic responses (biofeedback), it has been shown that people may be able to control responses formerly regarded as involuntary, such as heart rate and blood pressure.

The autonomic nervous system is further divided into the sympathetic and parasympathetic divisions. Broadly, the functions of the two divisions of the autonomic system are antagonistic. Activation of the sympathetic system tends to increase expenditure of body energy, whereas activation of the parasympathetic system tends to decrease expenditure of energy.

Activation of the sympathetic nerves of the autonomic nervous system tends to increase energy expenditure. Activation of the parasympathetic nerves tends to inhibit energy expenditure.

In effect, the sympathetic neurons act like an accelerator, whereas the parasympathetic neurons act like a brake. During stress, pain, emotional excitement, threat of injury or states of emergency, the neurons in the sympathetic system are activated and body resources are mobilized for "fight or flight". This activation causes dilation of the pupils, a rise in blood pressure, deeper respiration, increased heart rate and increased sweating, accompanied by inhibition of the parasympathetic system. The adrenal glands secrete adrenalin into the bloodsteam which in turn enhances the action of sympathetic neurons.

The parasympathetic nervous system tends to inhibit sweating, heart action and so on. It conserves, rather than mobilizes, energy resources. If you have nearly been hit by a car you have

Some of the functions performed by the autonomic nervous system. The two divisions, the sympathetic and parasympathetic, tend to be antagonistic in operation but there are many exceptions to this simplification.

PARASYMPATHETIC EFFECTS	TARGET ORGAN	SYMPATHETIC EFFECTS
constricts pupil	eye (pupil)	dilates pupil
stimulates salivary gland viscous secretion	salivary glands	stimulates salivary gland watery secretion
dilates blood vessels	blood vessels	constricts blood vessels
constricts respiratory passages	trachea and lungs	dilates respiratory passages
decreases heart rate	heart	increases heart rate
stimulates digestive activity	stomach and intestines	inhibits digestive activity
	adrenal gland	stimulates adrenalin secretion

felt the effects of the sympathetic system — your heart races, you sweat, your stomach feels like a rock. However, gradually you recover as your parasympathetic neurons steadily restore normality.

In addition to the electrochemical communication network of the nervous system (Chapter 1) there is a parallel *chemical* communication network (the enodcrine system) that operates by way of the blood system. The message units of this system are hormones. (see 9.4).

3.3 The central nervous system (CNS)

There are three major divisions of the central nervous system — the spinal cord, the sub-cortex and the cortex. The cortex is the outer layer of the brain.

The neurons of the central nervous system form a cohesive structure which floats in the cerebrospinal fluid (CSF) and is attached to the skull by fine fibrils. Within the central nervous system, the spinal cord includes the neurons housed in the bony casing of the spinal vertebrae, while the cortical level is represented by the neurons of the outer layers of the cerebral hemispheres. The subcortical level includes those cells of the CNS which lie above the spinal cord and below the cortex.

The cortex refers to the outer layers of the brain. The sub-cortex consists of the structures of the brain beneath the cortex but above the spinal cord.

3.4 The spinal cord

The spinal cord contains neurons which carry information to and from the higher brain regions. Information from receptors is passed to higher brain centres via spinal neurons. Information from the higher centres travels down the spinal neurons and is passed to the efferent neurons of the peripheral nervous system. For example, messages to "move the hand" or "lift the leg"

To experience a sensation neural information must reach the brain.

The simplest neural circuit is between a receptor, a neuron and an effector. This sort of circuit underlies simple spinal reflex responses such as the kick elicited by tapping the patellar tendon.

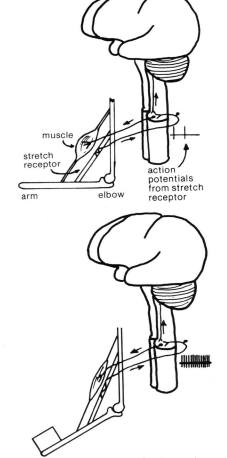

muscle

stretch
receptor

arm   elbow

action
potentials
from stretch
receptor

How a stretch reflex works. Increasing the load on the arm increases firing in the stretch receptors which in turn results in muscle cells being activated to compensate for the increased load.

travel from the brain via spinal neurons to the efferent neurons which then relay them to the effectors.

If the spinal cord is cut or damaged, a person no longer experiences any sensation originating from below the point of the break. This lack of sensation occurs because neural information that reaches the body receptors must pass to the higher brain levels before a sensation is felt. Voluntary movement of the limbs is not possible in such cases, since all messages concerning voluntary movement of body parts normally are passed to the spinal neurons from higher brain levels.

However, there are some simple neural pathways completed within the spinal cord, for example direct synapses between sensory (input) neurons and motor (output) neurons. In this case, information travels directly from the afferent neuron to the efferent neuron and the effector, and a motor response occurs. Such connections underlie what are referred to as *spinal reflex responses*.

Probably the most simple spinal reflex is the *stretch reflex*. In each skeletal muscle there are receptors responsive to the degree of muscle stretch. If the muscle stretch is increased, for example by an unexpected increased load on the arm, action potentials are initiated by the stretch receptors. The potentials travel down the axons of these stretch receptors to the spinal cord. There the stretch receptor axons synapse with spinal motoneurons, which emerge from the spinal cord and return to the muscle.

The action potentials from the stretch receptors increase the firing of the motoneurons, resulting in increased tension of the muscle to compensate for the new load. This increased tension decreases the stretch of the stretch receptor, reducing its firing and in turn reducing the need for additional muscle tension. This simple reflex is called a *monosynaptic reflex*, as only one synapse is involved. In normal people some information from the stretch receptor travels up the spinal cord to the brain. Therefore we feel the stimulus after the reflex response has occurred.

The stretch reflex is tested during a standard medical examination — the doctor taps our knee with a hammer. This suddenly stretches the muscles and they quickly compensate for the increased stretch which results in the knee-jerk. Spinal reflexes are innate in that their performance does not depend on past experience.

Although quadriplegics are incapable of voluntary movement, they do have spinal reflexes. In quadriplegics, vital cardiovascular and respiratory processes continue because the damage to the spinal cord is below the area where the relevant autonomic neurons leave the spinal cord.

Other, more complicated reflexes are also completed within the spinal cord but they involve a number of synapses. The reflexive withdrawal from a painful stimulus is one such *polysynaptic reflex*.

3.5 The brain

In evolutionary terms the brain consists of a primitive central core — the brain stem, the thalamus and the cerebellum. Around the thalamus there is a cluster of nuclei and interconnecting fibre tracts that were originally thought to be concerned primarily with processing information about smell. This group of structures is collectively referred to as the *limbic system*. The outer layer of the brain — the new brain or neocortex — has evolved upon the limbic system. Despite this evolutionary division, the various structures are interconnected in a complex fashion.

The primitive parts of the brain are the brain stem, thalamus and cerebellum. The newest part of the brain to evolve is the cortex.

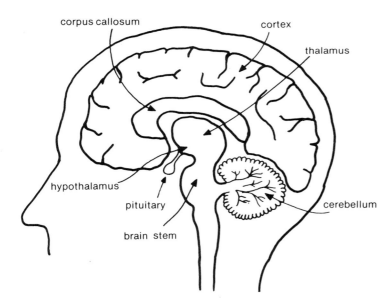

A simplified section through the middle of a human brain.

The brain stem forms a stalk which supports the other brain structures. It is made up of the following anatomical divisions — the *medulla*, the *pons*, the *mid-brain*, the *colliculi* and the *reticular formation*. The latter is a region of fairly densely packed neurons and nerve fibres, forming a "core" of the brain stem.

The brain stem contains ascending and descending fibres which transmit information to or from higher brain centres. There are also neurons within the brain stem which relay incoming information directly to motor efferents. These brain stem reflexes include sucking, swallowing, sneezing, coughing, yawning, breathing, and the control of blood pressure. That the reflexes are organized within the brain stem is demonstrated by their presence in children born without a cerebral cortex.

The central core of the brain stem is the reticular formation. It is important in the control of sleep, waking and many other functions.

The thalamus, which is located at the top of the brain stem, is a major relay station for sensory and motor information.

Not all reflexes are adaptive. Infant cot deaths may be due to inappropriate activation of a vestigial diving reflex (see also 6.5). The diving reflex is a complex pattern of responses including reduced heart rate and cessation of breathing. This reflex allows certain animals to dive to great depths and survive under water for considerable periods without air. It has been suggested that in newborn children some unusual stimuli may elicit this inappropriate reflex with fatal results.

The cells in the central part of the brain stem make up the *reticular formation*. This region receives input from all sensory systems and maintains a continuous barrage of impulses ascending to the cortex. The reticular formation is involved in the control of sleeping, waking and many other physiological and behavioural functions (see 6.8).

Located on top of the brain stem but still deep beneath the surface of the brain is a pair of football-shaped structures which form the *thalamus*. A major function of the thalamus is to relay information to and from the cortex. (The stippled area in the diagram shows where these fibres projecting to the cortex have been cut.) Many nuclei of the thalamus receive input from sensory afferent fibres and project it to the cortex. For example, the lateral geniculate nucleus receives input from the optic nerve and projects to the visual cortex.

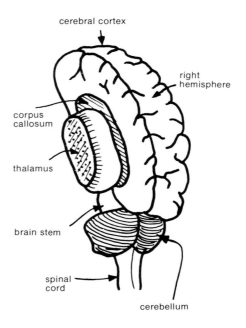

A view of the brain from behind, after the left hemisphere has been removed.

All senses except smell have relay centres in specific nuclei of the thalamus. Within these nuclei sensory information is modified before being relayed to the cortex. Some thalamic nuclei relay information from the cortex down through the spinal cord to the skeletal muscles. Other thalamic nuclei are involved in coordination of reflex movements of the eyeball and the pupillary reflex.

Surrounding the thalamus is a number of long nuclei. A group of these nuclei which form the *basal ganglia* are associated primarily with movement, whereas others appear to play a major role in emotional and regulatory behaviours. Such distinctions between psychological and motor responses are becoming increasingly blurred, as is indicated by terms like "psychomotor" epilepsy.

The basal ganglia, which are located around the thalamus, are important for the initiation and control of voluntary movement.

The basal ganglia include the caudate nucleus, the lentiform nuclei (together making up the corpus striatum), the claustrum and the amygdaloid nuclei. These nuclei are important for the initiation and control of voluntary movement. Damage to the basal ganglia produces a behaviour pattern called *obstinate progression*. For example, walking movements will continue even when forward progress is prevented by an obstacle. In Parkinson's disease, those cells in the basal ganglia which use the transmitter dopamine are defective. People with Parkinson's disease have difficulty starting and stopping movements, and suffer both stiffness and tremor when the limb is at rest. These symptoms can usually be removed by treatment with drugs like L-dopa which enhance dopamine metabolism (see 11.8).

Another structure important for movement control is the *cerebellum*, which is situated on the top surface of the brain stem and below the cortex. The cerebellum acts to smooth and refine muscular action. The cerebellum works with information from equilibrium sensors (vestibular sensory system) and information concerning the position of limbs and the stretch of muscles. In addition, the cerebellum ensures that motor commands from higher centres are coordinated and result in well-regulated movement.

The cerebellum, which sits on top of the brain stem just behind the cerebral hemispheres, co-ordinates and refines complex patterns of movements.

There are an enormous number of muscles involved in even simple actions such as using a knife and fork, or walking. A professional card player can deal cards with exceptional speed and precision. This probably involves "reading off" a carefully prepared program of this action which is stored and refined by the cerebellar neurons.

People with damage to their cerebellum have overactive reflexes and disturbances of timing and coordination, particularly of rapid movements. For example, when reaching for a glass, if they do not reach in the correct direction, rather than making a minor correction, which people generally do automatically, these people repeatedly over-correct their movements, which often results in wild swinging movements.

The hypothalamus, which is generally considered to be part of the limbic system, is involved in regulatory mechanisms as well as autonomic and endocrine functions.

Situated in front of and slightly below the thalamus is the *hypothalamus*. This brain region is important in the regulation of glandular secretions, eating, drinking, sexual behaviour, emotional behaviour, and body temperature. The hypothalamus is unusual in that it manufactures chemicals (hormones) which are transmitted, via the bloodstream, to the adjacent pituitary gland. Hypothalamic hormones control the pituitary gland's manufacture of a number of hormones which are carried by the blood stream to control both the manufacture and release of the hormones of other glands (such as the release of the hormone adrenalin by the adrenal medulla). Thus the hypothalamus functions as an important link between the brain and the glandular effector system (see 9.4).

Questions

1 What constitutes the central nervous system.
2 In which direction do afferent neurons transmit information?
3 What are the main divisions of the peripheral nervous system?
4 Skeletal muscles are controlled by which set of nerves?
5 What does "autonomic" mean and why may it now be inappropriate?
6 What activates sympathetic nerves?
7 What effects do parasympathetic nerves have when they are activated?
8 What is the name of the fluid bathing the brain? To what use has it been put?
9 What is a spinal reflex?
10 What are the most primitive parts of the brain?
11 In evolutionary terms, what is the most recently developed part of the brain?
12 What function has been traditionally ascribed to the limbic system?
13 Name five reflexes organized in the brain stem.
14 What is the main sensory function of the thalamus?
15 The basal ganglia are important for the control of which behaviours?
16 Describe a characteristic disability produced by damage to the cerebellum.
17 Why is the hypothalamus unusual?

Further Readings

Barr, M.L. *The Human Nervous System: An Anatomical Viewpoint.* New York, Harper & Row. 1979.
Noback, C.R. and Demarest, R.J. *The Nervous System: Introduction and Review.* New York, McGraw-Hill. 1972.

4

Functional Anatomy of the Cortex

4.1 Introduction

The most conspicuous parts of the human brain are the two folded masses which together form the *cerebral hemispheres*. The two hemispheres are separated by a deep fissure running from front to back, beneath which they are connected by a bundle of fibres called the *corpus callosum*. The corpus callosum is the largest and most important of the connecting or commissural fibre systems of the brain.

Each hemisphere is approximately the size of a clenched fist. The average human brain has a volume of 1300 cm³ and weighs 1.4 kg. The values vary considerably but, above a certain lower limit, brain volume has no relation to intelligence. Each hemisphere is filled largely by message-carrying fibres. However, much of the work of the brain is done in the cells which form the outermost layers of the cerebral hemispheres. These layers are called the *cortex* (from the Greek word for bark).

The importance of the cortex is indicated by the fact that primitive organisms, such as fish and frogs, have no real cortex. As behavioural complexity increases, the size of the cortex increases correspondingly. The increased development of the cortex contrasts with other structures such as the cerebellum and the thalamus, which generally remain in proportion in cats, monkeys and humans.

The appearance of the cortex tends to change with the complexity of the organism. In primitive animals such as the rat the cortex is smooth, whereas in primates the cortex is convoluted with large folds (fissures) and ridges (gyri). The convolutions greatly increase the surface area of the cortex although much of it is hidden from view.

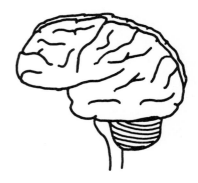

Illustration of the human brain as seen from the side.

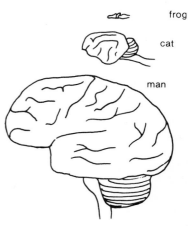

The relative sizes of cortex in frog, cat and man.

39

Many fissures may slightly differ from individual to individual but the large fissures are fairly constant. These main fissures are the central fissure and the lateral fissure, which facilitate the division of each hemisphere into four lobes — the frontal lobe, the parietal lobe, the temporal lobe, and the occipital lobe. These divisions simplify relating of brain function to cortical location.

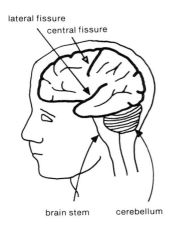
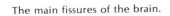

The main fissures of the brain.

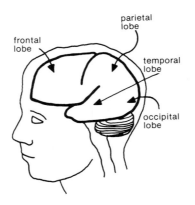

The lobes of the brain. Each hemisphere is divided into these four lobes.

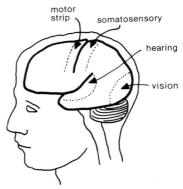

The main projection areas on the cortex for the major sensory systems.

4.2 Cortical regions involved in sensory function

All sensory systems have neural pathways which terminate in *sensory projection areas* of the cortex (also called cortical projection areas). This implies not a direct connection between receptors and the cortex but rather a sequence of neurons. The sensory projection areas of both hemispheres are generally of equal size.

The cortical projection areas are essential for the proper sensing of particular stimuli. Visual information projects to the occipital lobe, auditory information to the temporal lobe, somatosensory information (touch, pressure, etc.) to the parietal lobe.

Parts of each projection area appear to serve as primary areas (since damage to them leads to total loss of that sensation). Regions bordering each primary projection appear to serve an integrative function. For example, damage to the occipital lobes may result in some loss of vision although the eyes and optic

nerves are in perfect working order. Damage to regions bordering on the visual cortex results in normal visual sensation but
with deficits in *integrating* the visual sensation experienced.

Recent studies of people with damage to their visual cortex
have found that, if the damage is small, a small spot of blindness
— a scotoma — occurs in their visual field. If a light is flashed in
this spot when the eyes are fixed on a target, the person sees
nothing. However, if patients are forced to make judgements
about whether a line presented on this blind area is vertical or
horizontal, they perform significantly better than chance.

The reason seems to be that, rather than all the output from
the eye finding its way to the cerebral cortex, some fibres branch
to part of the brain stem (the superior colliculus). These fibres
remain unaffected by damage to the visual cortex. It appears that,
when forced, a person can draw upon this brain stem information. The results support the view that, while for conscious
perception the appropriate part of the cortex needs to be intact,
rudimentary sensory functioning can continue without it.

4.3 Cortical regions involved in motor responses

Electrical stimulation of the cortex in awake humans undergoing
neurosurgery has revealed regions of the cortex having detailed
control of skeletal muscles. The "motor strip" is 2–3 cm wide
and is located in front of the central fissure. Within the motor
strip there are large cells with long axons which fire off instructions to the skeletal muscles via the spinal cord. The motor
cortex of the *left* hemisphere controls muscles in the right side of
the body and vice versa.

The spatial representation of the skeletal muscle groups along
the motor strip is fairly consistent from person to person. Thus
Penfield and Rasmussen were able to map which parts of the
motor strip control particular body muscles.

Electrical stimulation of the strip of cortex behind the central
fissure yields reports of touch or tingling sensations in specific
parts of the body. The strip is the main cortical projection area
for somatosensory sensations, and Penfield and Rasmussen were
also able to map where on the surface of the brain particular parts
of the body are represented.

The motor and somatosensory maps have two features in
common. First, there is virtually a *total cross-over* of somatosensory input and motor output. In each case the left hemisphere
receives information about the right side of the body and controls movements of limbs on the right side. This is consistent
with evidence of people who suffer strokes restricted to one
hemisphere. Subsequent paralysis (motor area damage) or

The region of the cortex involved in motor responding is the motor strip just in front of the central fissure.

The left hemisphere controls movements of the right side of the body and vice versa.

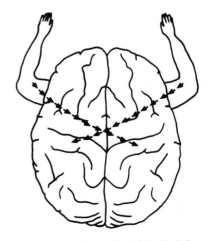

Sensory input from the left half of the body goes to the right half of the brain and vice versa.

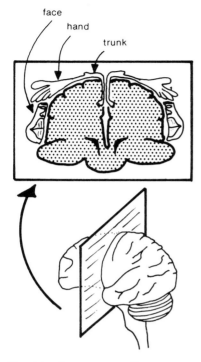

The strip of cortex controlling motor function is called the motor strip. It is about 3 cm wide and runs down both hemispheres. Various regions of the strip control movement of various parts of the body enabling 'maps' of function such as those in the upper half of the diagram.

Areas of the cortex not directly concerned with sensory or motor processes are called association areas.

A number of functions are not represented symmetrically in both hemispheres.

numbness (somatosensory area damage) is restricted to the side of the body opposite the brain damage. Second, in both the motor and somatosensory systems, the amount of cortex representing a particular region of the body is related to the precision with which we can manipulate that region, or to its tactile sensitivity. Consequently, the maps of body representation and muscle control are oddly distorted. For example, a large cortical area receives information from and controls the fingers, whereas a much smaller area of cortex represents the body trunk. A further example of this principle can be found in the pig, which has a disproportionately large cortical area related to the snout.

Parallel systems and parallel processing is a major theme of the neurosciences, and is exemplified by the motor system. The main motor strip of the cortex is part of the *pyramidal system*, which is important for the control of discrete limb movements. However, there is another motor control system — *the extra-pyramidal system* — which is largely independent of the pyramidal system. This system seems to be concerned primarily with movements involving both sides of the body, such as eye movements, neck movements and walking. For example, patients with damage to the pyramidal system are unable to use one side of their body for movements, such as kicking or stamping out a cigarette. However, some can walk, bow and kneel quite normally (responses controlled by the undamaged extra-pyramidal system). The extra-pyramidal motor system also regulates the level of background excitation or muscle tone. The rigidity and resting tremor of Parkinson's disease are examples of an extra-pyramidal system dysfunction (see 11.8).

4.4 Non-specific cortex (association areas)

Large areas of the cortex of humans are not directly concerned with sensory or motor processes. These regions, which are called non-specific cortex or association areas, integrate sensory input and motor output. The association areas are relatively small in primitive animals and relatively large in humans. In the rat most of the cerebral cortex is committed to sensory or motor processes, whereas in humans the total cortical area committed to primary sensory or motor functions is small. Further, our frontal, parietal and temporal lobes are more developed than those of more primitive species. Findings on the functioning of these association areas have been derived largely from studies of patients with localized brain damage. The extent to which perceptual learning and memory, motor learning and memory, and language are affected is related to the location and extent of damage to the cortical association areas. However, in humans, a number of association functions are not represented symmetrically in both hemispheres.

The sensory projection areas and motor areas of both hemispheres are virtually equal in area. However, the association areas show definite asymmetries. For example, the left hemisphere is dominant for *language* functions, almost irrespective of right or left-handedness. If the dominant hemisphere is destroyed before the age of approximately 11, the non-dominant hemisphere can assume the language functions, although the child may experience transient language difficulties. If the destruction occurs after age 11, the language loss is usually permanent.

The sensory projection areas of the cortex are the regions where the sensory pathways terminate.

The most conclusive demonstration of which hemisphere is dominant for language arises from the injection of the anaesthetic sodium amytal into one of the two carotid arteries. Each carotid artery supplies blood to only one hemisphere. If the injection causes muteness and other language errors, then it is concluded that the side injected is the dominant hemisphere.

Language functions are mainly controlled by the left hemisphere.

There have been many attempts to relate handedness (or sidedness) — the superiority of one hand (or side of the body) over the other — to cerebral dominance, with variable results. The variability is partly due to the inadequacy of the sidedness tests and the difficulty of adequately establishing cerebral dominance in non-brain-damaged people.

Handedness is genetically predisposed but can be modified by learning or brain damage. While 90% of the population is right-handed, left-handed people use their right hand much more often than right-handers use their left hand.

It is believed the superiority demonstrated in handedness may reflect a superiority of the cerebral hemisphere opposite to and controlling the superior hand. Liepmann suggested that the hemisphere controlling the superior hand was also the storehouse of the learning involved in motor skills. This implies that, when right-handed people are forced to use their left hand, they rely on information transmitted between the two hemispheres via the corpus callosum, from the "storehouse" hemisphere. This suggestion is consistent with the fact that paralysis of the right side (resulting from damage to the main controlling left hemisphere) results in left limbs which are unusually clumsy. This would be expected if the motor skills could not be transmitted across the corpus callosum.

4.5 Perceptual learning and memory disturbances

People with damage to the cortex just in front of the visual projection areas are still capable of visual sensations, but these sensations are not adequately integrated. Often patients will describe details of a figure presented to them, using certain details to guess the nature of the object. For example, one patient was shown a drawing of a pair of spectacles and was asked to name

Association areas around the visual cortex play a role in visual recognition.

Agnosia is a defect of visual recognition.

the object depicted. He responded, "a circle . . . another circle . . . a crosspiece — it's a bicycle." The general name for this type of perceptual disturbance is *agnosia* ("not knowing").

One variety of agnosia is the inability to recognize faces. One patient, with damage to the association areas of the parietal lobe, could describe all the markings and characteristics he saw when he looked into a mirror, but could not recognize his own face. Such cases reflect the problems of testing brain-damaged people. Are patients simply misunderstanding the questions, or do they have defective perceptual ability? Exhaustive individual testing is required to overcome these problems. In addition to these functions it now seems that areas of the parietal lobe may play an important part in directing eye movements and perhaps even directing attention.

Other cortical regions are critical for the integration or recognition of auditory and tactile material and they are centred around the major auditory and somatosensory projection areas.

4.6 Memory of skilled movements

The memory of skilled movements is affected by damage to the association areas around the motor strip.

Damage to association areas around the motor strip (in front of the central fissure) affects the memory of skilled movements. These patients are unable to remember or organize the sequence of movements making up particular skills. They can copy but cannot initiate the movement. The general name for this loss of motor memory is *apraxia*.

Apraxia is an inability to perform a sequence of movements.

Geschwind (1975, p.188) defines apraxias as "disorders of the execution of learned movement which cannot be accounted for by weakness, incoordination or sensory loss, or by incomprehension of or inattention to commands". He quotes the example of a patient who could carry out commands with his right hand (e.g. combing his hair or using a hammer), but when told to use his left hand made no response. He could copy the task with his left hand if the examiner performed it, but was apparently unable to integrate the movement sequence himself. The fact that he could copy the task with his left hand rules out weakness or incoordination. Further, as he could perform the task with his right hand, inattention, uncooperativeness or incomprehension were also ruled out.

4.7 Language disturbances

Aphasia is a loss of language ability.

Damage to association areas of the left temporal lobe produces language disturbances. A loss of language ability, due to brain damage, is called *aphasia*. Such disruptions are not primarily due to sensory or motor deficits, but to the inadequate handling of symbolic processes.

The two major cortical areas for language — Broca's area and Wernicke's area — are linked neurally. The location and extent of these areas has been the subject of dispute, and they do not have definite anatomical boundaries. Damage to these areas produces gradients of language loss.

Broca's area is at the base of, and just in front of, the central fissure. If it is damaged, disturbances of speech production result. These patients have great difficulty in speaking, and what speech they have is emitted slowly, with great effort and poor articulation. Some may have only a one-word vocabulary, and few can produce whole sentences. In addition, a similar disability usually occurs in their written language. However, they generally *comprehend* both spoken and written language.

The language loss produced by damage to Broca's area is not due simply to paralysis or muscular problems — patients can often sing the tune of a melody using "la-la". The essential deficit is one of integration because the neural machinery that integrates language production is damaged. It may be that Broca's area governs the transformation of language into speech or writing.

Wernicke's area is a region in the left temporal lobe, below the lateral fissure and adjacent to the primary projection area for hearing. Damage to this area results in the inability to understand both speech and writing. Speech and writing are produced effortlessly but are essentially meaningless — a scrambled sequence of meaningless, inappropriate and often unintelligible words and non-words. Interestingly, the basic grammatical skeleton appears preserved but there is a lack of denotation. Wernicke's area seems to govern the recognition and synthesis of language patterns.

There are close neural connections between Wernicke's area and Broca's area. Geschwind believes that the act of speaking involves the formulation of a concept into an auditory form in Wernicke's area, and then relaying it to Broca's area where the language is put into the complex programming of the speech organs.

There have been recent attempts to relate reading disabilities (*dyslexia*) and brain dysfunction. Certainly some cases of dyslexia are attributable to brain dysfunction, but reading is a complex task in which many functions such as eye movements and systematic scanning have to be integrated. Problems in any one of these areas could result in poor reading ability.

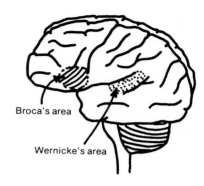

A side view of the left hemisphere showing the two major areas involved in the control of language function.

Language production is disrupted by damage to Broca's area. Language comprehension is disrupted by damage to Wernicke's area.

Dyslexia is reading disability. It is not simply related to brain dysfunction.

4.8 Language association areas in the non-dominant hemisphere

Language functions appear to be controlled by association areas in the left hemisphere of the brain. This raises a question about

The capabilities of the right hemisphere have been explored in patients in which fibres joining the hemispheres (the corpus callosum) are cut.

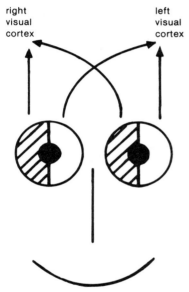

Front view of the eyes showing that the striped regions project to the same hemisphere.

the function of the comparable regions of the right hemisphere. It was once thought that the right hemisphere was relatively unimportant since massive strokes to the right hemisphere had very little effect on language. However, the significance of the association areas in the right hemisphere is now becoming evident. The evidence is derived largely from the study of patients with damage to the corpus callosum, so that their two hemispheres function relatively independently. Other evidence has come from patients with massive damage to their left (dominant) hemisphere, so that they are totally without language functions (global aphasics).

In the mid-1950s, Sperry showed that, if the fibres joining the two hemispheres of monkeys are cut, each half of the brain functions independently of the other. In 1961 Bogen and Vogel showed that this "split-brain" operation in humans relieved some cases of severe epilepsy. Initially there appeared to be remarkably few side-effects. However, specialized tests revealed many functional disturbances.

Stimuli presented to a restricted part of the visual field reach only one hemisphere (see 5.3). Since the corpus callosum is cut in these patients this information is not transferred to the other hemisphere. If a written command is presented to the right half of the visual field so that the message is conveyed only to the left hemisphere, the patient can *say* what the command is and respond accordingly. If the command is presented to the left half of the visual field so that it goes to the right hemisphere (the non-dominant hemisphere for language), the patient cannot say what the word is. However, there is evidence that the right hemisphere does recognize the word. For example, if the written word "key" is presented to the right hemisphere only, the patient cannot say the word but can pick a key out of an array of objects with his left hand (which is controlled by the right hemisphere).

For some skills the right hemisphere is superior to the left. Spatial abilities (such as copying block-designs) and musical abilities are apparently more disrupted by damage to the right hemisphere than to the left.

Thus the right hemisphere is not illiterate. Furthermore, it has been found that people who have lost the use of the association areas in their left (dominant) hemisphere, have considerable residual semantic and syntactic capacities which can be realized through response systems other than speech. Gazzaniga found that such patients can perform many language operations using only their right hemisphere and, for example, could quickly learn "same or different" judgements. The discovery of the full capacity of the right hemisphere awaits the ingenuity of those testing it.

4.9 The frontal lobes

The two frontal lobes constitute approximately 25% of brain volume, yet the functions of this massive amount of brain remain obscure. The frontal lobes were once believed to be the seat of intelligence, since the most intelligent animals appear to have the largest frontal lobes. Recent evidence suggests, however, that the role played by the frontal lobes is considerably more complex.

The frontal lobes have a role in attention, intellective abilities and personality.

In the early 1930s, Jacobsen removed both frontal lobes from the brains of a group of monkeys. After they had recovered from the operation they were subjected to a number of behavioural tests. The monkeys were found to perform particularly poorly on a delayed response task. Each monkey was shown a piece of food which was then hidden under one of two cups; after a short delay the animal had to select that cup. A correct response yielded the food. Since the monkeys without frontal lobes performed poorly on this task, Jacobsen concluded that the frontal lobes were important for immediate memory. However, recent evidence suggests that this interpretation is not correct. If the monkeys were in darkness during the delay, their performance was near normal, suggesting that the frontal lobes play a role in attention or distractibility rather than immediate memory. This interpretation is consistent with the findings of research on human subjects with frontal lobe damage.

At a conference in 1935, Jacobsen described one monkey which, prior to ablation, would throw a temper-tantrum if it made an error. However after the frontal lobe ablation it accepted the errors without throwing tantrums. Jacobsen's description apparently prompted a Portuguese neurosurgeon, Moniz, to treat some of his more severely psychotic patients by frontal lobe surgery. A variety of frontal lobe surgical procedures, such as lobotomy, were widely used in psychiatry until about the mid-1950s (see 9.15 and 9.21).

Attempts to infer the function of the human frontal lobes from the testing of lobotomized psychiatric patients are of limited value due to the abnormal nature of the subjects prior to ablation. A more useful source of evidence comes from testing normal people who have accidentally suffered frontal lobe damage (for example, through war or car accidents). Post-operatively such people do not become imbeciles, hence it is unlikely that intelligence is localized in the frontal lobes. Generally, behavioural changes due to frontal lobe damage are subtle, affecting both intellectual behaviour and personality.

The classic example is of a man named Phineas Gage who, about 100 years ago, was using a crowbar to tamp down a gunpowder charge for an excavation. The powder accidentally exploded and the crowbar was driven through his skull. (The crowbar and skull are on display at Harvard Medical School.)

The accident almost completely removed both his frontal lobes. Gage survived the accident and soon resumed work. However major changes in his behaviour took place. Whereas prior to the accident he was an excellent and conscientious foreman, after the accident he became careless, slovenly, unreliable and easily distracted.

Studies like this, including those undertaken by Russian neurologist, Luria, of Russian soldiers who had suffered frontal lobe damage, provide further insight into the functions performed by this massive volume of neurons. The behaviour of patients with frontal lobe damage is generally stereotyped or perseverative. An example of perseveration is a patient who, when asked to successively subtract 7 from 100, responded 100, 93, 83, 73, 63, . . . It appears that these people find it difficult to let go of a concept once it is formed. Similar stereotyped behaviour is observed in monkeys following frontal lobe removal.

As was the case with lobotomized monkeys, humans with damage to the frontal lobes are easily distracted. This distractibility may be reflected in their response to tests of intellectual functioning, although overall intelligence test scores are typically unchanged. These patients also have difficulty explaining the meaning of complex material, or in picking out significant objects in a picture. Luria characterizes these difficulties as follows: "In normal subjects the derivation of the meaning of a picture develops because of well-structured analytic or synthetic activity. In frontal patients this derivation is disturbed by ancillary associations evoked by fragmentary observations." The thinking of these patients is often described as being very concrete — they have difficulty explaining the meaning of a metaphor and in perceiving object relations and analogies.

In addition to intellectual changes, subtle changes in personality often occur; for example, there is a tendency to become more extroverted, while exhibiting a lack of purpose or initiative.

Finally, the fact that the loss of the frontal lobes has no measurable effect on intelligence test scores may be due to the unreliability of the intelligence tests used. They may be neither measuring the correct things nor weighting various sub-tests appropriately.

4.10 Recovery of function

The exact relationship between brain damage and recovery of function is not clear. While some individuals may exhibit severe and permanent loss of behavioural function, others with apparently similar brain damage can recover a lost function after considerable re-training. If the conditions which determine whether or not recovery occurs could be clearly described, the whole area of rehabilitation after brain damage could be approached on a more scientific basis.

LeVere has argued against the widely held view that recovery of function depends upon other neural systems "taking over" the processing formerly done by the now non-functional neurons. Rather, he suggests that recovery occurs because a behaviour pattern may involve the operation of many parallel systems. Therefore, destruction of one area can leave the parallel systems to continue as normal. However, Gazzaniga's research suggests that, by appropriate manipulations of the encoding instructions and responses, it may be possible to "shunt around" a brain lesion. Furthermore recent histological experiments with animals have demonstrated a possible mechanism for the recovery of brain function following damage. It was found that neurons damaged by experimental lesions appear to regenerate nerve terminals. The process, *axonal sprouting*, results in the production of more nerve terminals than were present prior to neuron damage.

Questions

1 How are the two hemispheres of the brain interconnected?
2 Does man have the largest brain?
3 Does intelligence depend on brain size?
4 What are the four lobes of each hemisphere called?
5 What are the sensory projection areas of the cortex?
6 Where are they for vision, for touch, and for hearing?
7 Which part of the cortex controls motor responding?
8 Which hemisphere controls movements of the right side of the body?
9 Describe the principle apparently pertaining to the representation of body parts on the cerebral cortex.
10 What functions are the extra-pyramidal motor system concerned with?
11 How is evidence about the function of the association areas of the cortex obtained?
12 Which hemisphere is usually dominant for language?
13 What are the consequences of damage to visual association areas?
14 What is agnosia?
15 What are the consequences of damage to the association areas around the motor strip?
16 What is apraxia?
17 What is aphasia?
18 What are the two cortical regions important for language functions?
19 What are the different functions of Broca's area and Wernicke's area?
20 How can the abilities of the right hemisphere be studied?
22 Does the right hemisphere play a significant role?
22 Name two abilities affected by damage to the frontal lobes.

Further Readings

Blakemore, C. *Mechanics of the Mind*. Cambridge, Cambridge University Press. 1977.
Geschwind, N. Specialization of the human brain. *Scientific American*, 1979, **241** (3), 158–168.
Kolb, B. and Whishaw, I.Q. *Fundamentals of Human Neuropsychology*. San Francisco, Ca., W.H. Freeman. 1980.
Pincus, J.H. and Tucker, G.J. *Behavioural Neurology*. New York, Oxford University Press. 1974.
Walsh, K.W. *Neuropsychology: A Clinical Approach*. New York, Churchill Livingston. 1978.

5

Sensory Systems

5.1 General principles of neural coding

Our senses do not always accurately reflect the physical world. The information arriving at the brain is modified and transformed in distinctive ways, so that in many cases it bears only a tenuous relationship to the physical world.

In Chapter 1 we noted that a strong stimulus generally causes a nerve cell to fire at a higher rate than a weak stimulus does. However, during presentation of a prolonged intense stimulus, the firing rate is initially high but gradually decreases. This decrease in firing rate is called *adaptation*. Adaptation leads to ambiguity. A given firing rate could result from a weak stimulus which has just been presented, or from a strong stimulus which has been presented for a long time. All the brain receives is the given firing rate. In such situations we experience an illusion. A strong stimulus after a long time is perceived as less intense, although physically the stimulus has not changed. We all experience these illusions. During the first few minutes of a swim, the water feels cold but gradually seems to warm up. Our cold receptors are gradually adapting. Their firing rate decreases to a rate normally elicited by luke-warm water. Something like adaptation seems to occur in most sensory systems, with the possible exception of pain.

It has been suggested that if adaptation did not occur we would be constantly distracted by trivia. Some theorists even consider that the almost universal occurrence of adaptation reflects a basic principle of brain function. The nervous system downgrades the importance of maintained stimulation and increases the impact of information about changes in stimulation.

Adaptation is a gradual decrease in firing during prolonged stimulation.

The nervous system seems to enhance information about changes in stimulation.

51

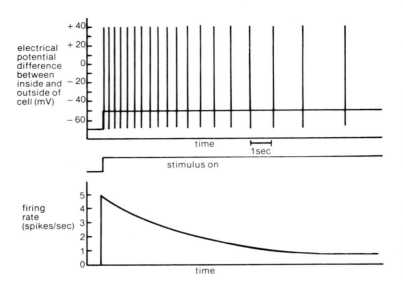

During prolonged stimulation firing rate decreases. This decrease in firing rate is called adaptation.

Certain aspects of neural coding are ultimately responsible for the lack of complete correspondence between the real world and our perception of it. The question of neural coding requires some consideration.

Information carried by the cells of the nervous system is coded in the form of action potentials that are essentially invariant in size and speed. Only the frequency of action potentials changes. The identity of action potentials for all cells raises two questions:

- How can the brain discriminate between different types of stimuli, such as sounds, colours and smells?
- How can neurons convey all the qualitative information in a particular stimulus to the brain? For example, in the case of visual stimulus, how do we experience its brightness, shape and colour?

These two questions may be reduced to the following:

- How does the brain distinguish differences between and within sensory systems?

In 1826 Müller tried to answer the first question in his doctrine of specific energies of nerves. Müller believed that a part of the mind called the *sensorium* (something like a little person in the head) did the ultimate sensing.

The sensorium was not directly aware of external objects but only of states of the sensory nerves — as Müller put it, the "energies" of these nerves. He observed that differences between senses depend on which nerve is stimulated, not on the source of stimulation. Müller argued that the receptors for each sense are usually only excited by the appropriate kind of stimulus, an "adequate" stimulus, such as light for the eye. Essentially, Müller's doctrine states that the interpretation of input is determined by the receptors from which the neural input comes. For example, the brain interprets certain impulses as visual, resulting in a light being seen, because the input to the central nervous system comes from receptors in the eye, not from receptors in any other sensory system. The emphasis is upon the place of reception.

Müller's doctrine appears to explain not only our lack of perceptual confusion in distinguishing between senses, but also the occurrence of occasional illusions. The sensorium knows only which sense organ is stimulated, not how. Hence we see light not because light enters the eye but because neurons in the optic nerve conduct information. The doctrine implies that, if we can excite the receptor by an unusual stimulus, the same sensation will result. This is in fact the case. Pressing the eyeball, an unusual stimulus, produces the same visual sensation as light, and electrical stimulation of the tongue gives the same taste sensation as salt.

Müller's doctrine has also a practical application. Some people lose the receptor hair cells in the inner ear and become totally deaf, although the neurons from the dead receptor cells still function normally. If these neurons could be activated by other means, the people should report hearing sounds. One method that has been used to activate the neurons is stimulation through electrodes. When the auditory nerves of totally deaf people are activated by electrical stimulation, they report hearing sounds. The technique of activating neurons in various parts of the nervous system by weak electrical current and observing the subject's responses has provided much information about the function of parts of the brain.

However, Müller's doctrine cannot account for our ability to distinguish between sensations within the one sensory system. To be consistent, it should imply that there are differences within a sensory system because different receptors are stimulated. For example, in vision there should be different receptors for colour, brightness and shape. The place of stimulation is important in some respects, but it is inadequate for conveying all the information within a sensory system. "Place" theories cannot explain how we can see the difference between a red triangle and a green square when they are presented successively to exactly the same receptors.

To answer the question of coding within each sensory system, it is necessary to look at how specific aspects of a stimulus affect the rate of firing of individual nerve cells.

How does the brain distinguish between senses and within a sense if all input is in the form of identical action potentials? Müller's answer: you see a light because the input comes from the optic nerve.

*Generally, increasing intensity
increases firing rate and in addition
activates less sensitive cells.*

*Decreases in firing rate can be as
informative as increases.*

*With two simultaneous stimuli, neural
interaction can occur, modifying the
neural coding of each stimulus.*

Some general principles are common to most sensory systems:

1. Increasing the intensity of stimulation usually increases firing rate. Also, as intensity is increased, less sensitive cells are brought into operation, so that increasing stimulus intensity generally both increases firing rate and activates more cells.

2. Lack of action potentials or inhibition can be just as meaningful as a burst of impulses. An important feature of the activity of most nerve cells is that they may fire without any synaptic input from other cells. For example, neurons in the optic nerve randomly initiate action potentials even in complete darkness. This random firing is called spontaneous activity. The presentation of some stimuli may increase the spontaneous firing rate, whereas other stimuli may decrease it. The brain derives information about the latter stimuli when cells, which normally fire at a certain rate, become suddenly silent during stimulation.

3. One significant advance in the understanding of the problem of neural coding has been the finding that, when two or more stimuli are presented simultaneously, there can be neural interaction between the cells sending information about each. The interaction modifies the pattern of neural firing produced by the presentation of each stimulus alone. The particular firing rate elicited in a cell in the visual system by a small grey patch can be changed depending on whether the patch is presented on a black or white background.

Some researchers have claimed that neural interaction explains the perceptual phenomenon of simultaneous brightness contrast. Whether or not that explanation is true, it is clear that because of neural interaction the general questions asked about coding represent an oversimplification. In real life we rarely see

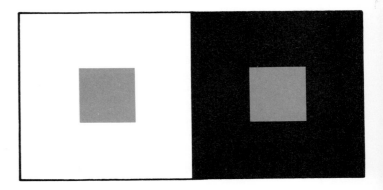

The central grey squares are physically identical. They do not appear so. This perceptual illusion is called simultaneous brightness contrast.

one colour over the whole visual field, or hear a single pure tone. Rather we see different colours side by side, and hear different tones simultaneously, so that the coding of each stimulus will depend on the characteristics of concurrent adjacent stimulation.

5.2 Vision: light and the eye

When we look at an object, light is reflected from that object to the back of our eyes. Visible light falls within a narrow range of the entire spectrum of electromagnetic waves. For our purposes the waves vary mainly in amplitude (size) and wavelength (distance from one peak to another). If the wavelengths are too short or too long, we experience nothing, although the physical stimulus continues to reach our receptors. The wavelengths of visible light range from about 400 to about 700 nanometres (or 700 nm; where 1 nm $= 10^{-9}$ m).

White light contains a combination of different wavelengths. If white light is passed through a prism, the prism bends short wavelengths more than long wavelengths so that the white light is split into its components. Adding all the wavelengths of visible light yields white. Colour or hue is a subjective sensation we experience when our eyes are stimulated by various wavelengths under the appropriate conditions.

Visible light falls within a narrow range of the spectrum of electromagnetic radiation.

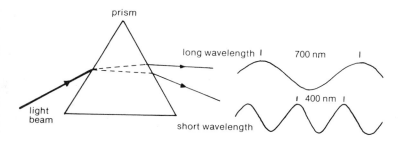

Light passed through a prism is broken into its constituent wavelengths.

The eyeball is roughly spherical and is made of tough fibrous tissue. Inside the eyeball is an elastic *lens*, and the remaining space is filled by jelly-like fluids. The transparent part at the front of the eyeball is the *cornea*. The *pupil* is formed by a small hole in the *iris*, the coloured circular muscle in the middle of the cornea.

The *retina* or the inner surface of the eyeball consists of thin layers of transparent photoreceptors and their associated nerve fibres. The *choroid coat* behind the retina is a layer of black cells which absorb stray light and supply blood to the retina. In some species, such as cats, the choroid layer is reflective, so their eyes appear to light up at night. The pupil in humans appears as a black hole because you are looking at the black choroid coat behind the retina.

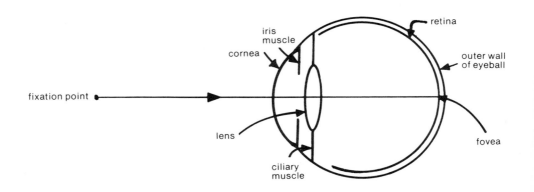

Horizontal cross-section through a human eye.

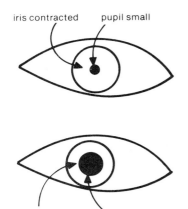

In dim illumination the iris muscle relaxes, reflexively.

Light enters the cornea, passes through the pupil and lens, and then forms an image on the retina at the back of the eye. The principle is identical to that of a camera. In both cases the size of the hole in a diaphragm controls the amount of light reaching the film or retina. In strong light the iris muscle contracts reflexively, reducing the total amount of light reaching the retina. In dim light the iris relaxes allowing the pupil to get larger and more light to reach the retina. Changes in pupil size have no effect on the size of the image formed on the retina. Changes in pupil size *alone* are not sufficient to permit good vision over the large range of light intensities experienced. Other structural and physiological characteristics of the visual system are important in enabling good vision over such a large range of intensities. These characteristics are discussed in later sections of this chapter.

The image on the retina is brought into focus partly by the cornea, which is like half a lens, and partly by the lens within the eyeball. The lens is supported around its outside diameter by the ciliary muscle. As the ciliary muscle expands and contracts, the lens bulges and flattens, thus changing its power. The change in power is called accommodation, permitting an easy change from viewing the TV screen across a room to reading the TV program in the hand. With increasing age, the lens hardens, the ciliary muscle also probably weakens, and it becomes difficult to focus on near objects.

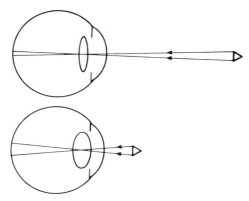

As objects approach, the lens expands to keep the image in focus on the retina.

5.3 The retina

The retina is made up of layers of cells. The outermost layer (i.e. most remote from the centre of the eye) consists of the photoreceptors. Synapsing on the photoreceptors are short afferents

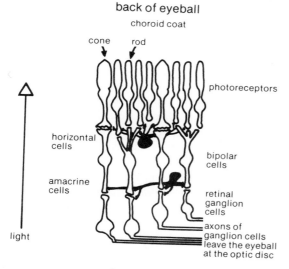

Schematic representation of the layers of the retina. All these cells are about as thick as a postage stamp.

called bipolar cells which, in turn, synapse on retinal ganglion cells. The axons of the retinal ganglion cells form a bundle called the optic nerve, which exits through a small opening at the back of the eyeball. The optic nerve projects mainly to the thalamus. Many neurons in the retina serve only to provide interconnections among other retinal cells. Horizontal and amacrine cells are the two types of interconnecting neurons in the retina. Because of these interconnections, one receptor can influence the activity of many nerve fibres to the brain.

Partly because of optics and partly because of neuroanatomy, there is almost complete cross-over in vision, as there is for the somatosensory input. If an object lies to the left of your fixation point, it projects to your right visual cortex and vice versa. The dividing line down each eye is a thin band which projects to both hemispheres.

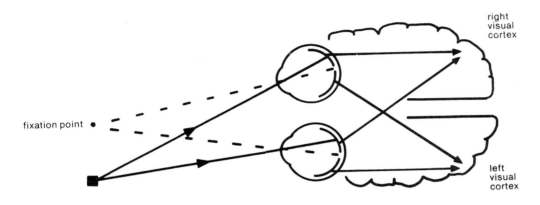

Partly because of optics and partly because of neuroanatomy there is almost complete cross-over in the visual system. Objects on the left of the observer project to the right visual cortex.

The retina contains two kinds of photoreceptors which, because of their characteristic shapes, are called *rods and cones*. The rods and cones are not equal in number, nor are they distributed uniformly on the retina. There are more rods (120,000,000) than there are cones (7,000,000) in an eye. The cones are concentrated in the *fovea*, a rod-free region of the retina directly behind the centre of the cornea. Whenever we look directly at an object, its image falls on the fovea, and it is here that visual acuity, the

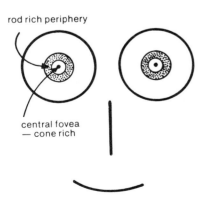

Front view of the eyes showing the most densely located regions of rod and cone receptors.

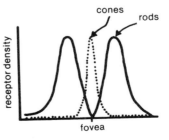

The relative density of receptors along a horizontal line drawn through the fovea.

ability to resolve detail, is greatest. Outside the fovea, cones are distributed with uniformly low density. Rods are most densely packed in a doughnut-shaped ring around the fovea. Outside this ring their density gradually decreases as distance from the fovea increases.

Another part of the retina is the *optic disc*, a hole in the eyeball where all the axons of the retinal ganglion cells leave the eyeball, forming the optic nerve. Since there are no photoreceptors at the optic disc, it is called the blind spot.

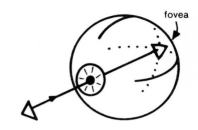

When an object is fixated an inverted image of it falls on the fovea.

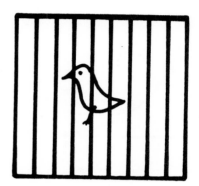

Demonstration of the blind spot. If you shut your left eye, stare at the cross and move the page toward you, at one point the bird in the cage will disappear. At that point the image of the bird is falling on the blind optic disc of your right eye, and as there are no photoreceptors at this point the bird is not seen.

5.4 The operation of the rod and cone systems

Towards the end of the last century, von Kries guessed correctly that the two kinds of photoreceptors function in a different yet complementary manner. The cone system functions at the high (*photopic*) levels of illumination that occur in daytime or under strong artificial lighting conditions. The cones permit resolution of fine detail and perception of colour. The rod system functions at low (*scotopic*) levels of illumination at which cones cannot function. The rod system is more sensitive than the cone system but is less efficient at resolving detail. One can see shapes at low light levels but cannot read a book. The two systems are complementary. The cone system yields high acuity but poor sensitivity, whereas the rod system yields poor acuity but high sensitivity. The cone system also detects differences in wavelength or colour.

We can consider an example of the different actions of the rods and cones. In the visual system, as in other sensory systems, prolonged intense stimulation reduces sensitivity. In vision this

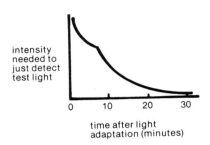

Recovery of sensitivity after exposure to strong light.

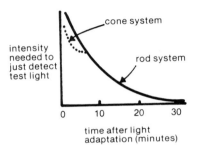

The previous graph is composed of two different functions.

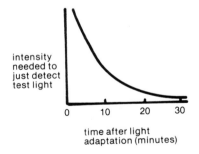

People with only rods in their retinas show no kink in the recovery curve.

Quanta are the bundles of energy which make up a light beam.

is called light adaptation. After exposure to strong light, the visual system takes time to recover its full sensitivity. This recovery from light adaptation is often called dark adaptation. One example of this recovery of sensitivity occurs when going from a bright street into a dim room. We cannot at first see much of the room since we have been light-adapted by the bright street. However, as we gradually recover from light adaptation, sensitivity increases. The process can be studied experimentally by exposing subjects to a bright light and then repeatedly testing their thresholds for visual stimulation, that is, the dimmest light they can detect as they recover from light adaptation.

Over time, sensitivity returns and their threshold decreases. There is a "kink" in this recovery curve after about 7 minutes. It is a "cross-over point" where the subject is shifting over from using the cone system to using the rod system to detect the test light. The kink occurs because the two systems recover at different rates. The cone system recovers quickly but never becomes highly sensitive. The rod system recovers more slowly but becomes extremely sensitive. That the lower branch of the curve is due to rod functioning is shown in experiments with people born without cones. Only the rod curve is obtained as sensitivity recovers.

5.5 The reception of light

In discussing the reception of light by photoreceptors, it is necessary to realize that light is made up of bundles of energy, each one of which is called a *photon* or a quantum (plural, quanta). Quanta can be thought of as the elements of a light beam, whereas the wave is a description of the whole beam. Increasing the intensity or amplitude of a light leads to an increase in the number of quanta it emits.

Once a photoreceptor absorbs one quantum, its resting potential changes. However, individual rods are more sensitive than individual cones and the rods and cones are "hooked up" differently. In the rod system, information from many photoreceptors converges onto one ganglion cell, whereas in the cone system the convergence is much less. The differences in receptor sensitivity and organization result in greater sensitivity for the rod system, which can detect light at much lower intensities of illumination than the cone system. This enhanced sensitivity is bought at the price of reduced acuity. At normal daylight and reading levels, we rely principally on the cone system since the rod system is saturated by the high intensities. The existence of the two different receptor systems permits efficient vision over a large range of illumination levels.

5.6 Light and colour

If we look at a coloured photograph of a spectrum in ordinary light, the various hues do not seem equally bright. The extreme wavelengths (700 nm, red and 400 nm, violet) do not appear as bright as those in the central medium-length greenish-yellow range of the spectrum. This brightness difference reflects the fact that the cone system is more sensitive to light of wavelengths around 555 nm and less sensitive to other wavelengths. If we take the photograph into a dark room, allow time for dark adaptation to occur, and look at the photograph again, we will observe two important changes. First, we will be able to see only colourless bands of greys, because the intensity of light is too low for the cone system to work and it is the cone system that is responsible for colour vision. However, unless it is extremely dark, there will be enough light for the rod system to function.

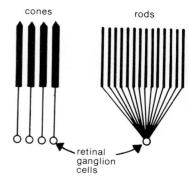

Typically, many rods converge on one ganglion cell. The convergence tends to be much less in the cone system.

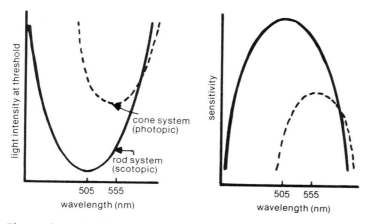

The graph on the left shows that the rod system has a lower threshold than the cone system for most wavelengths. In order to plot the relative spectral sensitivities the curves are simply inverted (lower threshold implies higher sensitivity).

The observation that objects lose colour at low light levels is to some extent difficult to understand. We normally think of colours as being part of the object. They are not. Objects only emit or reflect light of certain wavelengths. Colours are something we experience when stimulated by these wavelengths under the appropriate conditions, one of which is that the intensity of the light is high enough for proper functioning of the cone system. In the example above, or under night illumination, the objects still reflect the same wavelengths as they do during the day, but at night the intensities are low, the cone system does not operate, and therefore we cannot experience colours. Colour vision depends on the cone system.

We experience colours when the retinal cones are stimulated by light of appropriate wavelengths at fairly high intensity.

Returning to the example, the second change we will detect in the spectrum photograph is that the brightest part of the band of

The rod and cone systems have different spectral sensitivities.

Once any photoreceptor absorbs a quantum its resting potential changes.

greys we now see will shift from about 555 nm for the high illumination viewing to about 505 nm. This shift in brightness reflects the fact that the rod system is not only more sensitive overall than the cone system but that it is also most sensitive to shorter wavelengths than the cone system.

The difference in the spectral sensitivity of the two systems is useful in explaining many visual phenomena. For example, Purkinje noticed that, at twilight, blue objects seem to be brighter than red objects. The shift in relative brightness as intensity is reduced reflects the change from cone to rod vision, the rods being more sensitive to shorter (blue) wavelengths. This phenomenon is appropriately called the Purkinje shift. The intermediate light levels where both the rod and cone systems operate are sometimes called the mesopic range of intensities.

We need to consider now why cones can give rise to colour sensations but rods cannot. Every photoreceptor contains molecules of pigment which absorb quanta of light. Each of the 120,000,000 rods in the eye contains the pigment rhodopsin. Rhodopsin will absorb quanta of any wavelength but preferentially absorbs that at around 505 nm. Once a quantum has been absorbed by a pigment molecule, it has the same neural effect, regardless of its wavelength. Absorbing one quantum causes the same change in resting potential of the photoreceptor, regardless of the wavelength of that quantum. Consequently, a rod cannot convey information about what wavelength quantum it has absorbed. If 50 quanta are absorbed by a number of rods, the only information available to the brain is that 50 quanta have been absorbed. They could have originated from light of any wavelength.

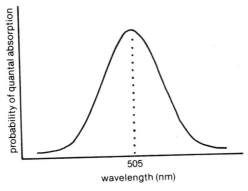

Probability of quantal absorption by rhodopsin for light of varying wavelength.

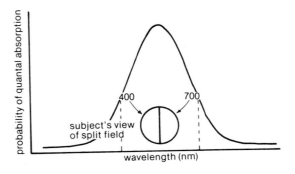

Lights of different wavelengths can cause the same number of quanta to be absorbed by rhodopsin.

For simplicity, assume we are testing a person with no retinal cones. Such an individual is referred to as a rod monochromat. We set up an experiment so that we can present to that person light of different wavelengths and intensity. If we shine a light of 700 nm on half a small split field, this will cause the rods to absorb perhaps 5000 quanta. If we shine another light of 400 nm next to it and adjust its intensity appropriately so as to also cause 5000 quanta to be absorbed by the rods, the only information available to the subject's brain is that 5000 quanta have been absorbed in each half. The two lights are not distinguishable to our subject. Since our subject cannot make wavelength discriminations, different wavelengths appear similar, presumably like greys of varying brightness as in a black-and-white TV picture. People with normal colour vision become similarly unable to make wavelength discriminations when the level of illumination is so low that only their rods can work.

If two different stimuli cause the same number of quanta to be absorbed, then the brain will receive the same message about both stimuli and the stimuli will therefore appear to be identical.

5.7 Colour vision

How do cones allow us to see colours? A cone is like a rod in that once a quantum has been absorbed, the cone cannot signal information about the wavelength of the quantum absorbed. However, while there is only one type of rod there are three types of cones. The pigment in some cones "prefers" quanta of short wavelengths (440 nm, "blue" cones), the pigment in others "prefers" quanta of intermediate wavelengths (535 nm, "green" cones), and the pigment in a third group "prefers" quanta of long wavelength (570 nm, "red" cones). Light of each wavelength causes a unique *pattern of absorption* by the three types of cone. For example, light of 490 nm will cause most absorption by the blue cones, less by the green cones, and very little by the red cones.

There is only one type of rod but there are three cone types.

It is the unique pattern of absorption by the three cone types which distinguishes between wavelengths and permits colour vision.

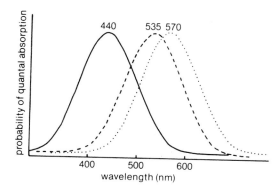

The probability of quantal absorption for the three cone types in the human retina.

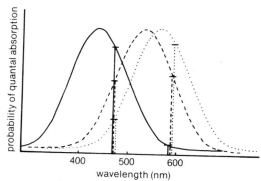

A light of 470 nm wavelength causes a pattern of absorption by the three cone types (vertical bars) that is totally different from the pattern of absorption for a 590 nm light.

Light of each wavelength causes a unique pattern of absorption by the three cone types. Therefore, information about wavelength is preserved and the cones mediate colour vision.

Consider a person with normal colour vision on the task we gave the rod monochromat. If illumination levels are high enough to activate the cone system, the 400 nm patch will cause a particular pattern of absorption in the three cone types. The adjacent 700 nm patch will cause a different pattern of absorption. No intensity adjustments can make the two patches match. Normal people will always be able to discriminate between them.

About 180 years ago Thomas Young suggested that colour vision is caused by three cone types in the retina, since by superimposing lights of three primary colours, it is possible to produce any hue. Helmholtz modified the theory and it became known as the Young–Helmholtz trichromatic theory of colour vision. This theory has since been found to be remarkably accurate. That there are three cone types in the human retina is shown by three independent sources of evidence.

Perhaps the most conclusive demonstration of the existence of three cone types comes from passing light through individual cone cells in the human retina and measuring the absorption of light of each wavelength. As the wavelength of the light is changed, the amount of light absorbed by the cone is measured. When this is done for many different cones, it is apparent that there are only three cone types in the human retina. Confirmation also comes from neural recordings of individual cone cells, and also from ingenious psychophysical experiments devised by Rushton. Cats and dogs seem to have two cone types. One species of turtle has five cone types. Its receptors would enable it to make wavelength discriminations impossible for humans.

The Young–Helmholtz theory is also useful in explaining the facts of additive colour mixture. If a pure light of wavelength 550 nm is observed, it will cause approximately equal absorption by the red and green cones and very little, if any, by the blue cones. If the pattern of absorption could be produced in another way, then its perceived colour should be indistinguishable from that of the 550 nm light. A similar pattern of absorption can in fact be produced by superimposing 535 and 570 nm lights. The additive mixture is indistinguishable from the single 550 nm wavelength. Similarly, the pattern of absorption produced by any single wavelength can also be achieved by the superimposition of three primary wavelengths, and the resultant colour appears similar.

The trichromatic theory accounts for many facts of colour blindness, since the three main types of colour blindness each correspond roughly to the absence of one of the cone types. If there are only two cone types present, then many wavelengths will cause the same pattern of absorption and the person cannot discriminate between them.

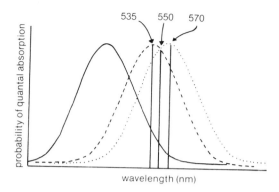

Additive colour mixture. There are different ways of producing the same pattern of quantal absorption.

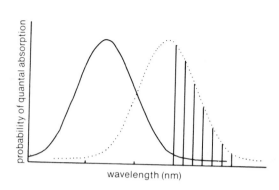

People with only two cone types cannot discriminate between many wavelengths (vertical lines) because all these stimuli cause similar patterns of absorption — much absorption by one cone type and very little by the other.

However, there are also many phenomena of colour vision for which the trichromatic theory cannot account adequately. In the 1870s Ewald Hering based a theory of colour vision on phenomena associated with complementary colours; that is, two colours which when mixed yield grey. One such phenomenon is successive colour contrast or negative after-images. If you stare hard at a glowing yellow light bulb and then look at a blank wall, you will see an after-image of the bulb coloured blue, the complementary of yellow. Red and green are also complementary colours.

In view of this phenomena, Hering proposed that there were three opponent processes in the visual system, a red–green opponent process, a yellow–blue opponent process, and a black–white opponent process. When a neutral grey stimulus is presented, these processes are in balance, and the perception corresponding to this equilibrium condition is grey. Stimulation by red upsets the balance and the perception corresponding to this out-of-balance condition is red. Prolonged stimulation by red will fatigue the red part of the red–green process. After this fatigue, presentation of a grey stimulus does not exactly restore the equilibrium condition. The red process is still fatigued, and so the green process slightly predominates, with the result that the grey stimulus takes on a green tinge, a green after-image.

Although Hering was not explicit about the "processes", there is now some evidence that the opponent-process concept is one way of describing how wavelength information is transmitted from the retina to the brain.

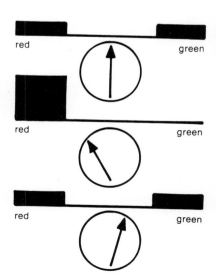

Representation of Hering's opponent process theory of colour vision.

5.8 The neural coding of wavelength

In 1966 De Valois recorded action potentials from single neurons in the lateral geniculate nucleus of the thalamus, the main relay station between the eye and the cortex.

Macaque monkeys were used because his behavioural experiments had shown that the spectral sensitivity curves of macaque monkeys were virtually identical to those of humans. De Valois chose to study only those neurons in the lateral geniculate nucleus which were spontaneously active, that is, which fired even when no light stimulus was present. For each neuron De Valois successively presented lights of various wavelengths and recorded how the firing of the cell was affected by each wavelength.

He found that the cells could be divided into three categories. Cells in the first category increased their firing when the retina was stimulated by intense long 570 nm light (red), but were inhibited if the wavelength was about 535 nm (green). Cells in the second category were excited by long wavelength light (570 nm) and inhibited by short wavelength light (450 nm). Cells in the third category were not dependent on wavelength. Firing increased for white light, decreasing as the light intensity decreased. In each category other cells were found showing the reverse pattern. For example, a cell would be inhibited by long wavelengths and excited by short wavelengths. As Hering predicted, each category of cells behaved in an opponent-process fashion.

In summary, the two most important theories of colour vision, which were developed in the 19th century, were not clearly confirmed until the 20th century. Remarkably, both seem to be fairly accurate descriptions of different aspects of colour vision. The Young–Helmholtz Trichromatic Theory describes the types of receptors, and Hering's Opponent-Process Theory provides an account of the way information from the three receptor types is transmitted to the brain.

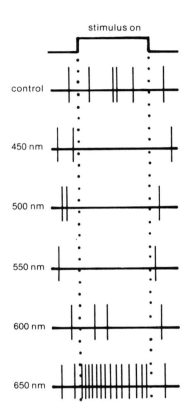

Each line shows the response of the same cell to light of different wavelengths. The cell's firing is reduced (inhibited) by short wavelength light and increased (facilitated) by long wavelength light.

5.9 The neural coding of contours

A contour can be defined as a change in the gradient of illumination. The diagram shows the type of graph we would obtain if we used a photometer to measure light intensity at successive points across a white bar on a black background. Each point represents the intensity of light at the particular spot shown on the stimulus, directly above. The contours occur whenever there is a change in the gradient of illumination. Psychologists and physiologists have concentrated on the manner in which such simple stimuli are coded neurally, the assumption being that more complex stimuli, such as letters, are simply combinations of elementary line stimuli.

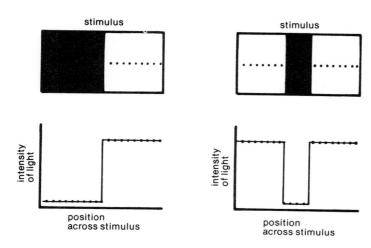

Graphs of light intensity at various positions across two stimuli. The change in intensity is called a contour.

One of the first and most important principles of the neural coding of contour has emerged from studies of the visual system of the horseshoe crab, *Limulus*. Limulus has a compound eye, like that of a fly, composed of many individual receptor cells. Each receptor cell has its own "private line" to the brain, its own afferent fibre. However, the afferent fibres are interconnected by laterally spreading branches. Hartline and Ratliff and their students have studied the way this eye codes information about light. The diagram on page 68 summarizes some of their more important results. Each row shows recordings of action potentials in the fibre from receptor D and the effect on the firing of fibre D by presentation of various stimuli.

If receptor D alone is illuminated by a weak spot of light, its firing rate increases slightly. If the light intensity is increased, the firing rate also increases. Within limits the firing rate is proportional to stimulus intensity. In the remaining rows the stimulation of D is maintained at the high level but other receptors are stimulated as well. Row 4 shows that if, in addition to stimulating the receptor D, the immediately adjacent receptors (C and E) are also stimulated, the firing rate of fibre D decreases. The firing rate of fibre D has been inhibited by the simultaneous stimulation of C and E. The laterally interconnecting fibres exert an inhibitory influence. Hartline and Ratliff called this phenomenon *lateral inhibition*, and they correctly reasoned that fibre D must also be exerting inhibition on its neighbours.

Lateral inhibition is mutual, so that the firing in any fibre can be reduced either by decreasing the intensity of the stimulus or by stimulating the adjacent photoreceptors simultaneously. In either case the information reaching the brain will be identical.

How are contours coded by simple eyes? In the horseshoe crab, neighbouring receptors can inhibit each other. As a result of mutual lateral inhibition, information about contours is enhanced.

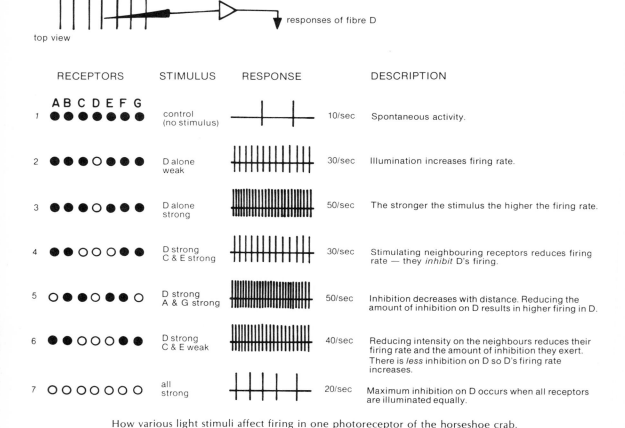

How various light stimuli affect firing in one photoreceptor of the horseshoe crab.

Increasing inhibition lowers firing rate, while decreasing inhibition increases firing rate.

Rows 5 and 6 show that the amount of lateral inhibition depends also upon the proximity of the neighbouring receptors being stimulated. Stimulating distant receptors causes little inhibition. Stimulating all receptors uniformly results in the greatest inhibition of a particular fibre (row 7).

Hartline and Ratliff proceeded to determine what happens if the Limulus eye is stimulated by a gradient of illumination ranging from black through grey rather than by simple spots of light. By recording from a single cell and moving the pattern across the eye in steps, they were able to deduce what they would have found had they been able to record from many receptors simultaneously.

Consider a row of receptors 1–22 activated by a stimulus ranging from black through grey to white. The lower graph shows the firing rate of the various cells. Receptors stimulated by the black region (1–5) receive little illumination and hence fire at a fairly low rate, thus exerting little mutual inhibition. However, cell 6, close to the change in stimulus from black to grey, will be subject to more inhibition than cell 3, because the receptors to one side (7, 8, 9) are being stimulated by the higher intensity grey, thus firing more, and exerting more inhibition on 6 than is exerted on cell 3 by its neighbours. Thus the firing of cell 6 will be lower than the firing of cell 3, because 6 is receiving more inhibition than 3. At the other extreme, cells 20, 21 and 22 are all strongly stimulated by the white. Hence they fire at a high rate and also exert considerable mutual inhibition between themselves. However, receptor 16, near the border between grey and white, will receive less inhibition from its neighbours (cells 14 and 15) which are stimulated by the lower intensity grey. Since it receives less inhibition, the firing rate in cell 16 can reach a higher level than cells 20, 21 and 22.

Thus, mutual lateral inhibition enhances information about changes in the gradient of illumination, the contour. Hartline and Ratliff have provided further evidence of the importance of lateral inhibition by demonstrating lack of "contour enhancement" in an experiment in which they physically prevented the inhibition from neighbouring receptors. The neural recordings faithfully reflected the stimulus intensity with no contour enhancement at the edges.

In the human retina there are many laterally interconnecting cells which probably behave in a similar manner. When humans view gradients of illumination, in appropriate conditions they report seeing a white band where the white changes to grey, and a black band where the grey changes to black. These bands are called Mach bands, and their appearance is consistent with the view that lateral inhibitory mechanisms operate in the human visual system.

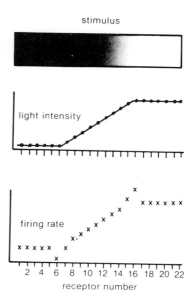

As a result of lateral inhibition the changes in the gradient of illumination — the contours — are enhanced.

Removal of inhibition can cause increased firing. This is called disinhibition.

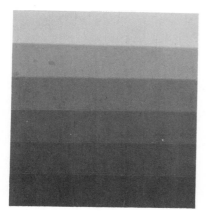

Each strip is a uniform grey but takes on a fluted appearance due to its neighbours. Some hold that the illusion occurs because of lateral inhibition: the lighter side of each border causes a higher firing rate which in turn exerts inhibition on cells being stimulated by the adjacent darker side. The increased inhibition lowers their firing rate — consistent with the stimulus close to the border being even darker than it really is. To demonstrate that this appearance of fluting is not due to some defect in the photographic or printing process, cover all the stips except one with white paper. Observe that each strip is uniformly bright across its width when viewed on its own.

As discussed previously, there are 5 main cell types in the human retina. The photoreceptors, the rods and cones, convert light to neural energy, which is transmitted as changes in resting potential and conducted to the bipolar cells and then to the ganglion cells. The other two cell types, the horizontal and amacrine cells, provide lateral connections across the retina. The details of information transmission within the retina are still not fully understood, but it is clear that a ganglion cell typically receives input from a group of photoreceptors occupying a small area of the retina.

5.10 Feature detection

In recent years much has been discovered about neural events in the sensory systems of cats and monkeys. Since psychophysical data on humans are usually consistent with the results obtained with these animals, it is reasonable to suppose that human sensory systems function similarly.

Recordings of activity in single neurons in the visual system have shown that these neurons integrate and process visual information in different distinct ways. The processing tends to be more complex at higher levels in the visual system, but the result is that different neurons in the visual cortex respond to different "features" of a visual stimulus, features such as line orientation, line width, and direction of line movement.

Neurons in the visual system respond selectively to various features of the stimulus.

Neurons in the visual system are clearly *not* like wires joining each photoreceptor to a neuron in the visual cortex.

How can we study the neural coding of visual information? Perhaps the most useful technique is as follows. The animal is anaesthetized and its head is fixed in a stereotaxic device (see 2.3) in front of a projector screen. A microelectrode is inserted into some part of the visual pathway to detect the action potentials

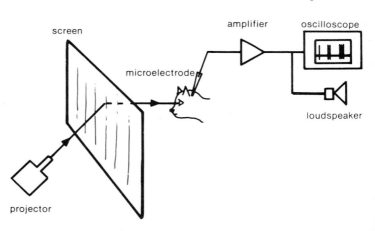

Experimental set-up to record neural responses to visual stimuli.

from a single neuron. Spots, bars and various stationary or moving patterns can be projected on the screen and thus on the animal's retina. We can then identify which stimuli affect a particular cell's firing rate. There are two ways in which a neuron's firing can be affected by the stimulus. It can either increase or decrease. These effects are referred to as excitation or inhibition respectively. Once a cell has been studied, the microelectrode may be advanced to detect impulses from another neuron, and the procedure repeated.

5.11 Retinal ganglion cells

Since a retinal ganglion cell receives its input indirectly from many photoreceptors, we would expect its firing rate to be affected by light falling on any of the photoreceptors. In fact, as Kuffler established, the firing rate of most retinal ganglion cells can be affected by a small spot of light directed anywhere within a retinal area of a few square millimetres. This region of the retina is called the *receptive field* of the cell.

The response of the cell depends on where the spot is directed within the receptive field. For some cells, spots anywhere in the central region cause increased firing (excitation), but if the spot is directed a little away from the central region, it causes the cell to decrease firing (inhibition). Kuffler called the regions ON and OFF regions respectively, and found that about half the retinal ganglion cells from which he recorded had ON centres and OFF

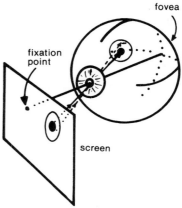

Spots of light shone in an area of the screen (and hence an area of the retina) can affect the firing of one ganglion cell. This area is called the receptive field of the cell.

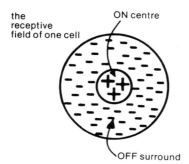

The effect of the light spot on the cell's activity depends on its location in the receptive field of the cell. In this example, spots shone on the centre cause excitation (+), whereas spots on the surround cause inhibition (−).

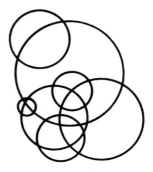

Each circle represents the receptive field of a different retinal ganglion cell. There is considerable overlap and variation in size.

surrounds. The surround forms a doughnut-shaped region around the central area. The other half of the ganglion cells had the reverse organization, OFF centres and ON surrounds.

Kuffler demonstrated that the strongest ON response was obtained by enlarging the spot so that it filled the ON area. This indicates spatial summation of excitation. Similarly, the strongest OFF response occurred when the light filled the OFF area, indicating spatial summation of inhibition. If the entire receptive field of the cell is uniformly illuminated, the excitatory input to the ganglion cell is often cancelled by the inhibitory input. Thus the ON and OFF areas are mutually antagonistic. However, if a bar or edge is appropriately located on the receptive field, the entire ON area, but not the entire OFF area, is stimulated. The

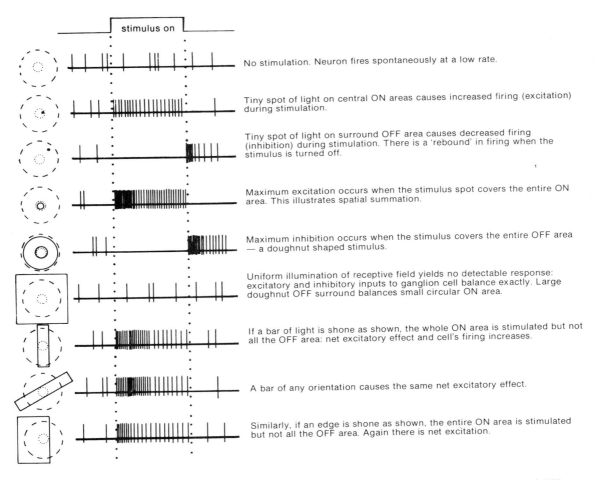

The effect of various stimuli on the firing of one typical retinal ganglion cell. The cell has an ON centre and OFF surround.

result is a net excitatory effect. Some theorists consider retinal ganglion cells to be spot detectors or edge detectors, responding best to the discrete stimuli rather than to diffuse illumination.

The receptive fields of retinal ganglion cells tend to be circular, to vary considerably in size, and to overlap one another. This overlap occurs because each photoreceptor can send information via the interconnecting horizontal and amacrine cells to many different retinal ganglion cells.

Single ganglion cells can have their firing affected by stimuli presented anywhere in a given *area* of the retina. Thus, the information transmitted from the retina to the brain concerns areas, not just points. In addition, the responses of retinal ganglion cells are selective — even at the retina some stimuli are better than others.

The antagonistic interaction between the centre and surround of a ganglion cell is important in explaining how the visual system can operate over an enormous range of intensities. Barlow and Levick studied this antagonistic interaction in individual retinal ganglion cells. If the receptive field of the cell is entirely illuminated by light at a fairly low level, the excitation and inhibition tend to cancel each other out, so there is no change in the cell's firing. If the weak uniform illumination is left on and a small weak spot is superimposed on this weak background, and the spot is positioned to fall on the excitatory region of the receptive field, then there is an increase in the cell's firing. This spot has "upset the balance" between excitation and inhibition so that excitation predominates and the cell's firing increases. Repeating this experiment on the same cell at much higher levels of illumination yields the same result. Intense uniform illumination yields no change in firing because the excitation and inhibition again cancel each other out. If the strong uniform illumination is left on and a small weak spot is superimposed on this strong background, then there is an increase in the cell's firing. Once again, this superimposed spot has "upset the balance" between excitation and inhibition. These important experiments show that sensitivity is maintained over a large range of illumination intensities by means of the antagonism between excitation and inhibition.

The next relay station along the visual pathway is the lateral geniculate nucleus of the thalamus. The responses of neurons in this nucleus resemble the responses of retinal ganglion cells. Their receptive fields are circular with antagonistic interaction between centre and surround. However, there is a considerable difference between the responses of neurons in the lateral geniculate and neurons in the visual projection areas of the cortex.

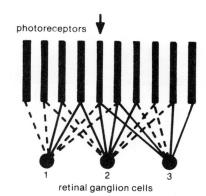

Each photoreceptor in the retina can send information to many different retinal ganglion cells. The information may be excitatory (solid lines) or inhibitory (dotted lines). In this way stimulation of one photoreceptor (arrow) may excite one retinal ganglion cell and inhibit another.

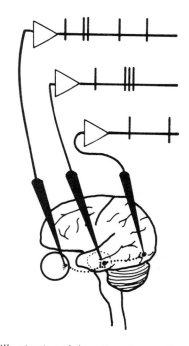

Illumination of the retina changes the firing rate of retinal ganglion cells, as well as that of cells in the lateral geniculate nucleus of the thalamus and cells in the visual cortex.

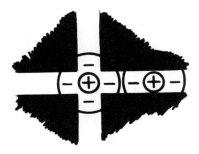

Consider two ON-centre receptive fields, one centre on a white intersection, the other centred on a straight white line. The former will be excited because its ON region is stimulated by white, but it will also receive inhibition from the four OFF regions stimulated. On the other hand, an ON-centre cell centred on a straight arm will be excited as much as the first cell but receive *less* inhibition because only two OFF regions are stimulated. The net effect will be that the first cell fires at a lower rate than the second cell and a lower firing rate is consistent with a weaker stimulus — hence the dark spots.

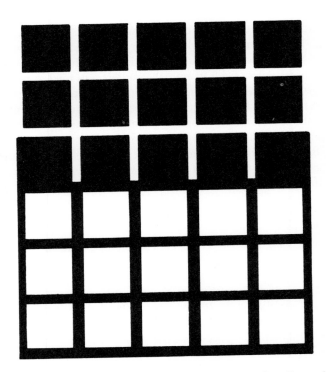

This illusion (the Hermann grid) has been said to show the effects of inhibition in the human visual system. If you stare at any white intersection the surrounding intersections appear to have dark spots on them. The spots disappear when fixated. The reverse occurs in the lower half of the figure.

5.12 Neural coding in the visual cortex

Hubel and Wiesel, two students of Kuffler, have studied the way in which visual information is coded in the visual cortex. They found a considerable range in the level of response complexity. The simplest cortical cells have ON and OFF areas which can be mapped using points of light. However, the ON and OFF areas of visual cortical cells are very rarely circular, concentric regions. Instead, they tend to be elongated into rectangular areas.

For many visual cortical cells, the "best" stimulus is a white line on a black background, for other cells it is a black line on a

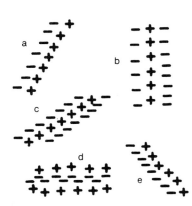

Examples of the type of receptive fields of the simplest visual cortical cells. Each letter represents the receptive field for a different cell.

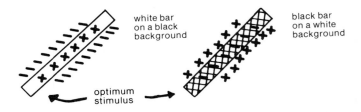

Elongated receptive fields of visual cortical cells are optimally stimulated by lines or bars.

white background, and for others it is a border between black and white. In each case the stimulus line or edge must be at a particular orientation and at a specific retinal location. If the location and orientation are correct, the stimulus elicits a large increase in the firing rate of the cell. If the orientation of the bar is changed, then the firing rate decreases. It is as if the cell is "tuned" to detect a line at one particular orientation. Different visual cortical cells are tuned to lines of different orientations. For this reason, visual cortical cells are often referred to as orientation detectors.

Different visual cortical neurons are tuned to detect lines at different orientations.

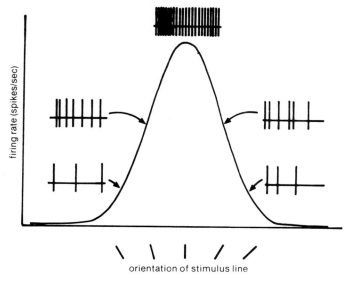

The firing rate in one cell to lines at different orientations. The cell fires maximally when the line is vertical and fires less as the bar is tilted away from this orientation. Other cells 'prefer' different orientations.

In addition to the simple cells there are other cells which are more specific in terms of the stimulus preferred. For example, in a complex cell, maximal firing may be produced by a stimulus line at a particular orientation and with a particular direction of movement. Consequently, this type of complex cell is often referred to as a motion detector or direction-selective neuron. Other cells, "hypercomplex" cells, are still more specific, firing maximally to a stimulus of particular orientation, direction of movement and length.

Hubel and Wiesel tried to explain the different levels of complexity by a hierarchical theory. They proposed that in the visual cortex the response of more complex cells is built up from the combination of receptive fields of simpler cells. If a simple cortical cell receives input from five lateral geniculate cells with receptive fields arranged one above the other, the shape of the simple cortical cell receptive field will be elongated and the optimum stimulus will be a vertical line.

Hubel and Wiesel suggested a serial 'hierarchical' theory to explain the increasing complexity of response of visual cortical neurons.

If a complex cell receives input from a number of similar simple cells, then it could respond to a bar of the appropriate orientation moving over a larger region of the retina. Similarly, the response of hypercomplex cells could be built up from the combination of a number of complex cells.

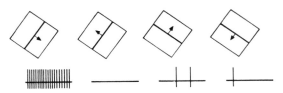

A complex cell 'preferring' a line of a particular orientation moving in a particular direction.

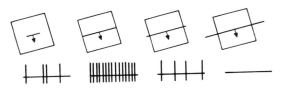

A hypercomplex cell. To elicit the maximal firing rate the stimulus must have a particular orientation, be moving in a particular direction and be of a particular length. If the line is too long the cell's firing rate decreases.

While this hierarchical theory is simple and elegant, recent evidence suggests it is not entirely accurate. For example, according to the theory it should take longer for a stimulus to elicit firing in a hypercomplex cell than in a simple cell because it must take time for the serial processing to occur. But this is not the case. Other evidence also argues against serial processing of visual information and instead suggests parallel processing.

Hubel and Wiesel also observed that about 80% of the visual cortical cells of the cat were binocular in that they were maximally activated by identical stimulation of the two eyes. The receptive fields of many cells were identical in location and shape in the two eyes, whereas other cells displayed small differences or disparities in the two fields. It is thought that these latter "disparity detectors" may underlie stereopsis, which is the cue to the depth perception that occurs when two eyes are used. Stimulus colour has also been shown to be an important property for some cells.

Hubel and Wiesel identified certain structural correlates of their physiological responses. If an electrode was inserted perpendicularly into the cortex, all cells picked up along the electrode track appeared to prefer the same orientation. Cells in other adjacent tracks preferred different orientations. Initially it seemed that the cells were organized in thin columns for each orientation. However, recent evidence suggests columns for a specific orientation are joined together to follow a wavy path

Recent evidence suggests that neural processing in the visual cortex is parallel, not serial.

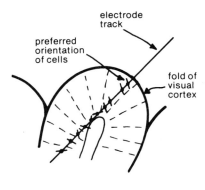

Cells in columns perpendicular to the surface of the cortex prefer lines of the same direction.

through the cortex. The anatomical organization of the visual cortex apparently reflects the different functions of various cell types.

5.13 Recent developments — the W, X, Y systems

Since the mid-1960s, researchers have re-examined Kuffler's original classification of retinal ganglion cells and have shown that there are three types of retinal ganglion cells called W, X (sustained cells) and Y (transient cells). The labels W, X and Y refer to the speed of conduction, W being the slowest and Y being the fastest.

There are three types of retinal ganglion cells which transmit information at different rates.

Y-type retinal ganglion cells (transient cells) have concentric ON–OFF (or OFF–ON) organization, but they respond mainly at the onset or offset of a maintained stimulus. They generally have large receptive fields distributed uniformly over the retina. Their thick axons enable them to relay information quickly. Axons of Y-cells branch so that, in addition to sending information to the visual cortex via the lateral geniculate nucleus of the thalamus, these cells also send a branch down to a region of the mid-brain called the superior colliculus, which is involved in eye movements. It is thought that Y-type cells are involved in "blind-sight" (Chapter 4). Complex visual cortical cells apparently receive much of their input from the fast Y-type retinal ganglion cells via Y-type lateral geniculate nucleus cells. This explains their shorter latency. Apparently Y-cells are more concerned with motion or change than with detail. For Y-type cells the focus of the stimulus is not critical.

Y-cells — fast conducting, large receptive fields, transient response at stimulus onset.

X-type retinal ganglion cells also display concentric ON–OFF (or OFF–ON) organization, but their firing tends to be maintained during a maintained stimulus. On average they have smaller receptive fields, concentrated around the fovea. Their axons are not as thick as those of Y-cells, so they conduct information more slowly. All X-cells project via the lateral geniculate nucleus to the visual cortex where they apparently synapse on simple and hypercomplex cells. For X-cells the stimulus focus is critical. They seem to be more concerned with detail.

X-cells — slower conducting, small receptive fields, sustained response during the stimulus.

W-type retinal ganglion cells do not have concentric ON–OFF organization. They are small cells with thin axons which, consequently, transmit information slowly. Apparently they project to the brain stem where, according to one hypothesis, they control pupillary responses. Recently it has been found that branches of W-cells also project to the visual cortex, via the lateral geniculate nucleus of the thalamus.

W-cells — very slow conducting, possibly controlling pupillary responses.

It now appears that, instead of one serial visual system as suggested by the hierarchical theory, there are two or three parallel visual systems. The transient or Y-system detects information about movement and relays it quickly to the brain stem.

The information causes our eyes to turn to look at the new or moving object with our foveas, using our "detail-detecting" X-cells (or sustained cells). Whether this simplification is adequate remains to be seen, but it does seem to be consistent with the differences between the X and Y-cells mentioned above.

There seem to be three parallel visual systems.

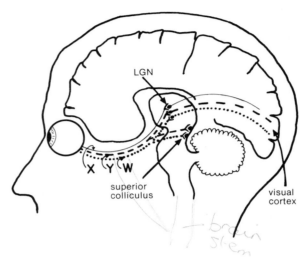

The three cell types all project to the visual cortex. The Y and W systems also project to the brain stem.

5.14 The relation between physiology and human perception

In summary, the evidence about the physiology of vision shows that the visual cortex is composed of cells that are maximally responsive to specific features of a stimulus. Much current research in perception is concerned with trying to explain human perceptual phenomena in terms of these findings in physiology. The following provides an example of this approach.

During intense maintained stimulation, neurons typically undergo adaptation — their firing rate decreases. When this maintained stimulus is turned off, the adapted neurons take some time to recover. Psychologists have tried to use this selective adaptation to study feature detection. Human observers report that, after prolonged visual stimulation by bars moving in one direction, stationary stimuli seem to be moving in the opposite direction. This is called the motion after-effect, and it has been suggested that it may be due to selective adaptation of motion-detecting neurons. In 1963, Barlow and Hill found some cells in the rabbit's visual system which responded maximally to bars moving in one direction, but whose firing was unaffected by bars moving in the opposite direction. Other neurons showed the reverse pattern. They suggested that the perception of motion may be due to the difference in firing rate between these two opposite types of motion detector. When the stimulus consists of bars moving to the left, then the leftward motion detectors will be activated, whereas the rightward motion detectors will not. The brain will receive the information that the leftwards detectors are firing more than the rightwards detectors and so the perception will be of movement to the left. Apparently simple, but vital, assumptions like this are needed to bridge the gap between brain and perception.

Barlow and Hill observed that, if the stimulus is maintained, these motion-detecting neurons show gradual adaptation. For example, as the bars move to the left, initially the leftwards detectors fire at a high rate, but as the stimulus continues their firing diminishes. When the stimulus is stopped after this prolonged stimulation, then the activity of these leftward detector cells falls below their spontaneous rate and only gradually returns. During this recovery time, therefore, the rightward motion detectors would be firing (spontaneously) at a higher rate than the leftward motion detectors. The brain would be receiving information that the rightwards detectors were firing more than the leftwards ones — as if a real stimulus was moving to the right. This is the motion after-effect: after prolonged viewing of leftwards moving bars a stationary grating appears to be moving to the right.

Other after-effects may be due to adaptation of more specifically tuned cells; for example, those tuned to orientation and colour. The explanations suggested are similar to that outlined above. Initially there is some balance and the stimulus is correctly perceived. Fatigue upsets this balance so that the same stimulus is incorrectly perceived. All these adaptations probably derive from Hering's explanation of negative after-images and Müller's doctrine.

The perceptual motion after-effect may be due to fatigue of motion detectors in the visual system.

5.15 The effect of early visual experience

In cats, early experience can affect the functioning of the visual system. In normal adult cats there seem to be approximately equal numbers of orientation detectors for all orientations. Developmental influences on the orientation detectors have been studied by rearing kittens from birth until about seven weeks in darkness, except for one hour a day during which they are placed in a lighted cylinder containing only vertical stripes.

Raising cats in the "all vertical" visual environment results in a dramatic change in the orientation preference of cells in the visual cortex. Most cells prefer vertical lines, whereas few that prefer horizontal lines are found. Apparently, the early visual experience permanently modifies the orientation preference of

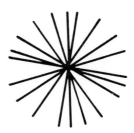

One way of representing the orientation preferences of many visual cortical cells in the one cat has been to superimpose lines at the optimal orientation for each cell. In normal cats the typical pattern is for equal numbers of cells at all orientations.

After restricting the visual experience of young kittens to vertical lines, all the cortical cells 'preferred' lines around the experienced orientation.

The characteristics of visual cortical cells can be altered by early visual experience.

the cells. In behavioural tests as adults, the cats appear to be blind to contours in the "deprived" orientation. For example, a cat that has received only vertical line stimulation will play with vertically waved rods but ignore horizontally waved rods.

Other more controlled techniques of selective contour exposure have been used. The cat can wear goggles with vertical stripes on them so that no matter how it tilts its head the lines on the retina are always vertical. This technique circumvents several of the objections to the cylinder-rearing technique which have recently been advanced.

In cats permanent modification occurs only if the selective visual exposure is given between about three and twelve weeks. Similarly, reversal of the effects is apparently only effective during the same critical period. These "plastic" changes in the functional organization of the visual system have attracted considerable attention as a possible model for understanding the neural changes that occur during learning.

It appears that the human visual system is also modifiable in a similar way. Astigmatism, a mis-shaping of the lens, so that contours in one orientation are blurred, once detected, can be optically corrected, resulting in substantial improvement in the subject's acuity for the blurred orientation. However, some "residual" astigmatism remains. It seems that the earlier astigmatism deprives the person of experiencing contours in one orientation, in a manner similar to that in which the cats in the cylinder are deprived. In humans, too, the deprivation has permanent neural consequences. Recent studies also suggest that there is a critical period in humans for the development of these pathologies.

5.16 Hearing and sound

Sound is a propagated pressure wave.

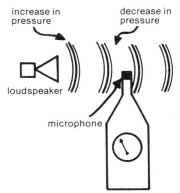

A microphone can measure the changes in air pressure produced by a loudspeaker.

If a kitchen fork is hit on a table, the fork prongs move back and forth (or oscillate) and a pinging sound is heard. The prongs alternately compress air particles and then reduce the pressure on them. A pressure wave is produced that moves away from the prongs. The pressure wave propagated in the air is detected as sound. The same thing occurs with a loudspeaker. The cone moves in and out, alternately compressing and reducing pressure on the air particles in front of the cone. A microphone can be used to measure the changes in air pressure occurring at a point in front of a loudspeaker, and these changes can be shown graphically. This particular pressure waveform may be described mathematically as a sine function, and so the sound is called a sine wave or a pure tone.

Varying the rate of oscillation alters the frequency of the tone. Frequency refers to the number of vibrations occurring in one second and is measured in Hertz (Hz). Increasing the frequency changes the waveform. The number of cycles per second increases, but the height or amplitude remains the same. The waveform on the left has a low frequency and that on the right a higher frequency. Low frequency tones are judged to have a "low" pitch and high frequency tones are judged to have a "high" pitch.

We can also vary the size or amplitude of the vibrations of a loudspeaker. The diagram shows the waveforms of a low amplitude and a high amplitude pure tone of one frequency. Pitch and loudness are psychological judgements. Frequency and amplitude are physical measurements.

Sound amplitude refers to the size or extent of the pressure wave variations.

Sound frequency is determined by how many of these variations occur in one second.

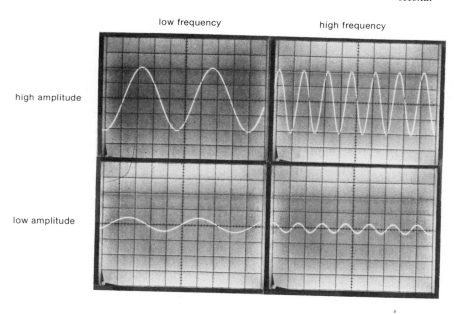

The effect of varying frequency and amplitude on the waveform of a pure tone.

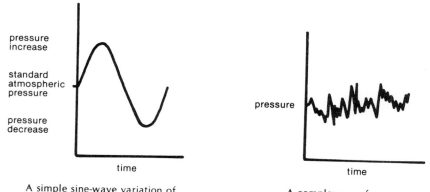

A simple sine-wave variation of pressure.

A complex waveform.

Speech is a complex waveform which can be analysed into individual pure tones.

Most sounds we hear have complex waveforms. Speech, for example, is a mixture of tones in which frequencies and amplitudes are changing quickly. Since complex waveforms can be analysed into combinations of sine waves, psychologists and physiologists have largely restricted their investigation to the use of sine waves or pure tones.

Young adults can hear tones of frequencies ranging from 20 Hz to 20,000 Hz. Middle C on a piano is 256 Hz and the highest C on a piano is 4096 Hz. The frequencies involved in speech range from about 100 Hz up to about 5000 Hz.

5.17 Anatomy of the hearing apparatus

Sound waves cause hair cells in the inner ear to bend. The bending produces changes in the resting potential of the hair cells, which in turn influence the firing rate of auditory afferent neurons.

The *cochlea*, which is the part of the inner ear concerned with hearing, is a coiled tube that looks like a snail shell. The cochlea consists of two tubes, one inside the other, similar to a car tyre. It is easier to understand how the cochlea works if we think of the cochlea uncoiled. If this could be done, it would be about 2.5 cm long. If we sliced along this uncoiled cochlea, we would find the two tubes. The inner tube is called the cochlear duct. If we

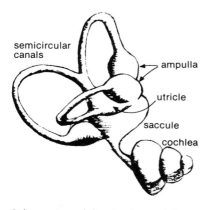

Side on view of the structures of the inner ear on the right side of the skull. The diameter of the semicircular canal is about 6 mm.

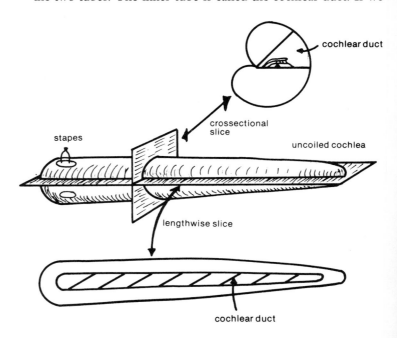

The cochlea uncoiled can be cut lengthwise (lower diagram) or crosswise (upper diagram). Both cuts show the 'inner tube' construction. The cochlear duct is the inner tube.

sliced across the uncoiled cochlea at any point, we would find
that the cochlear duct is triangular. The membrane making up
one side of this triangular inner tube is called the *basilar membrane*, and sitting on it are specialized cells some of which are
receptor hair cells similar to the hair cells in the vestibular system
(see 5.21). The auditory hair cells project into a jelly-like substance called the *tectorial membrane*.

*The basilar membrane is one side of
the inner tube of the cochlea. Along its
length are hair cells projecting into the
jelly-like tectorial membrane.*

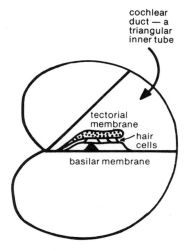

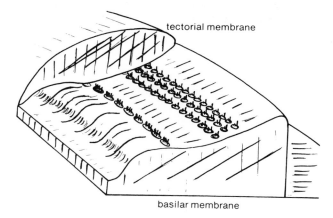

Enlarged view of a cross-section
through the cochlea.

Perspective view along a section of the basilar membrane. The tectorial
membrane has been removed from the nearer hair-cells.

The diagram shows a cross-section through the two tubes at
one point. The basilar membrane is running toward you and
away behind the page. There are regular rows of hair cells along
the basilar membrane. The close-up of one of these hair cells
shows its distinct "organ pipe" arrangement. The receptor hair

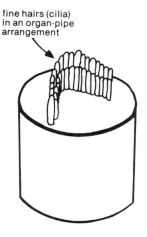

A representation of one hair-cell.

cells can be damaged or killed by intense or prolonged sounds and, like vestibular hair cells, they can also be damaged by high doses of certain antibiotic drugs. Once killed, the cells cannot regenerate. Surprisingly, we have only about 18,000 of them on each basilar membrane, compared with 127,000,000 photo-receptors in each eye.

How do the pressure waves in air bring about the deflection of the receptor cells on the basilar membrane? The pressure variations in air entering the external ear cause the delicate ear drum, or tympanic membrane, to move back and forth. The space behind the ear drum is filled with air, and almost opposite the ear drum on the other side of the air-filled cavity are the fluid-filled tubes of the inner ear, encased in bone.

Stretching across the air gap are three tiny, delicately suspended bones called *ossicles*. The last bone is called the *stapes*. The stapes looks like a stirrup, and the flat plate of the stirrup sits exactly in a hole in the bony casing of the cochlea.

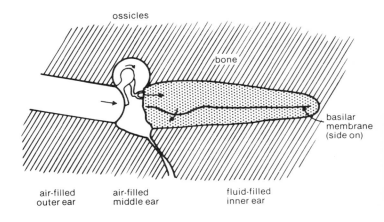

Operation of the ear.

5.18 Operation of the inner ear

Vibrations of the ear drum cause the ossicles to oscillate so that the stapes pumps the fluid in the cochlea at the same frequency as the tone driving the ear drum. This pumping causes the basilar membrane in the inner ear to move up and down with the same frequency as the tone. Because of the way the basilar membrane is constructed, it does not move uniformly along its length. Instead, the part of the basilar membrane which moves most depends upon the frequency of the tone.

The frequency of a tone is partly coded by which receptors are activated.

During stimulation by a tone, many points along the basilar membrane are moving up and down, but different tone frequencies result in some points moving up and down more than others. Low frequency tones cause most displacement of the basilar membrane far from the stapes, whereas high frequency tones cause most displacement close to the stapes. The diagram shows the amount of displacement along the basilar membrane for tones of increasing frequencies.

Variations in air pressure are conducted to the inner ear through the ear drum and then through three small bones in the middle ear, resulting in a pumping of the fluid in the inner ear. The pumping causes movement of the basilar membrane. With low frequency pure tones, that part of the basilar membrane furthest from the stapes moves most.

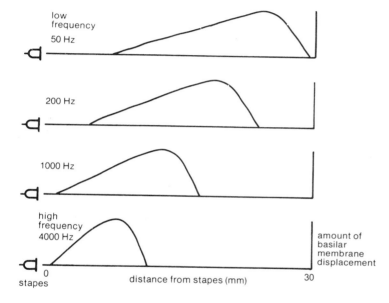

As the frequency of the tone increases, the region of maximum displacement shifts towards the stapes.

Each line is a graph of the amount of motion of the basilar membrane at various points along it. Each succeeding line shows that as the frequency of the tone increases the point of maximum movement shifts towards the stapes.

As the basilar membrane moves up and down, the hair cells on it are bent to and fro. The bending causes a change in their resting potential, and the firing rate of afferent neurons is changed. The hair cells in the region of the maximum basilar displacement are bent most. As a result the firing rate of neurons from this region will be most affected. In other words, the hair cells along the length of the basilar membrane are stimulated differently by tones of different frequencies. The frequency of a tone is coded by the place of maximum basilar membrane displacement.

How is the amplitude of a tone coded neurally? If we take a tone of a particular frequency and amplitude, it will cause a certain pattern of basilar membrane displacement, with maxi-

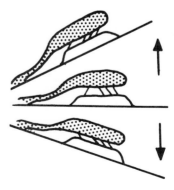

As the basilar membrane moves up and down at one point, the hair cells at that point are bent to and fro.

The amplitude of a tone is coded by the number of cells activated, and their firing rates.

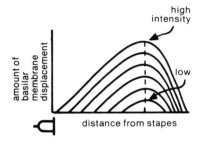

Varying the amplitude of a pure tone varies the amount of up and down movement of the basilar membrane.

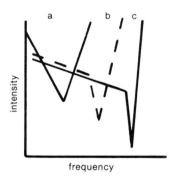

Each curve shows the limits of the combination of frequencies and intensities which cause increases in the firing rate of a neuron in the auditory nerve. The three curves are frequency tuning curves for three different cells.

mum displacement at one particular point. Increasing the amplitude of the tone causes greater displacement, so that the hair cells are bent more than for low amplitude tones, and more hair cells along the membrane are affected. Decreasing the amplitude of the tone reduces the amount of basilar membrane displacement, leaving the place of maximum displacement unaltered. At very low amplitudes, only a restricted region of the basilar membrane is affected and only a few hair cells are bent.

Recordings of action potentials in single neurons in the auditory nerve reflect this pattern. For high amplitude tones, a tone from a range of frequencies can cause an increase in that neuron's firing rate. As the amplitude decreases, the neuron is affected by tones within an increasingly narrow band of frequencies. Eventually, at threshold, the neuron is affected only by a tone of one frequency. The curve is a frequency tuning curve. At very low intensities each auditory afferent neuron is highly specific.

In summary, the frequency of sound is coded neurally by those groups of receptors and afferent neurons that are activated along the basilar membrane. Information about intensity or amplitude is given by the number of neurons that are activated and by their firing rate.

Sound can also be conducted to the inner ear by vibrations transmitted through the bones of your skull. The sound produced by clicking or grinding teeth is the result of bone conduction. When we speak, energy from the vocal cords reaches the basilar membrane both by conduction through the air and conduction through the bone. However, bone conduction transmits only low frequency sounds. If you listen to your voice recorded on a tape recorder, it sounds higher pitched than you expect. This is because it lacks much of the low frequency bone-conducted sound you usually hear when you speak.

Hearing loss can arise from damage to the neural machinery such as the receptor hair cells and afferent neurons, or from damage to the ear drum and ossicles. The latter kind of hearing loss is called conductive deafness and can be treated fairly simply, whereas the former kind, sensori-neural hearing loss, is virtually untreatable.

5.19 The neural coding of frequency

The basilar membrane oscillates at the same rate as the stimulating tone, and the hair cells on the basilar membrane are also bent back and forth at the same rate. If the frequency of the tone is low, around 100 Hz, recordings from primary auditory afferents show that many cells fire once per cycle, corresponding to the hair cell bending in an excitatory direction once during each cycle. However, as the frequency of the tone is increased, the cell is unable to follow the stimulus frequency exactly, since the maximum firing rate for a neuron is only about 1000 spikes per second. Nevertheless, careful analysis has shown that, even at frequencies much higher than 1000 Hz, frequency of cell firing is synchronized to the stimulus waveform.

In other words, a cell may fire on the first cycle of a 3000 Hz tone and then not respond for the next 10 cycles but then fire on the eleventh cycle and so on. A cell's firing can be "locked" or synchronized to the stimulus for frequencies as high as 4500 Hz and perhaps higher. It appears that the "locking" of cell firing to the stimulus waveform can be used by the brain to gain pitch information. Thus the coding of auditory frequency information is determined in multiple ways. Both the place of maximum basilar membrane stimulation and the rate of neural firing may convey information about stimulus frequency.

Since rate of firing gives information about frequencies, attempts have been made to overcome deafness by placing an electrode on the auditory nerve and delivering pulses of electrical stimulation to the healthly nerve fibres. This should cause neurons to fire synchronously with each pulse so that the brain should receive information consistent with a particular pitch. This has been done with deaf volunteers who appear to be able to discriminate between different rates. They can even identify a simple tune played by varying the rate of electrical stimulation. Such successes have led to attempts at presenting speech in terms of rates of impulses. There have been one or two claims of success, but so far the results are not particularly hopeful.

The broad pattern of basilar membrane displacement initially does not seem consistent with our acute ability to resolve the difference between two frequencies. Even at the periphery considerable sharpening has occurred. The tuning curves of primary auditory neurons should reflect the physical pattern of gradations in basilar membrane displacement. Instead, they are much sharper. The question has proved difficult to resolve because all the methods for physical measurement of the pattern of basilar membrane displacement involve some kind of interference with the cochlea, and the interference may contaminate the measures. Von Békésy has postulated that lateral inhibition sharpens the neural response to tones, but so far there is no satisfactory evidence of lateral inhibition in the cochlea. Research is currently directed at the sharpening mechanism, called the "second filter". It may be due to some unusual type of hair cell response.

The firing of auditory nerve fibres is locked or synchronized to the stimulus waveform for tones up to 4500 Hz.

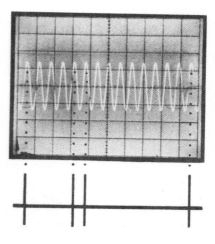

When an auditory nerve cell fires it is synchronized to the stimulus waveform.

5.20 Neural coding in the auditory cortex

In the auditory cortex, as in the visual cortex, individual neurons are tuned to, or prefer, specific aspects of the stimulus. Just as

Many auditory cortical cells prefer complex stimuli such as clicks and noise.

Some auditory cortical cells are spatially arranged so that cells preferring a given frequency are laid out in strips. This is referred to as tonotopic organization.

There may be two auditory systems.

many visual cortical cells cannot be activated by simple spots, many auditory cortical cells cannot be activated by pure tones but prefer complex stimuli such as clicks or noise. Brugge and Merzenich have made studies of the characteristics of auditory cortical neurons in monkeys. Some cells respond to pure tones and prefer a given frequency. These cells are arranged in strips, rather like the columns of cells preferring one orientation in vision.

In hearing, this structural correlate of frequency is called *tonotopic organization*, and its existence has been demonstrated over the entire auditory afferent pathway as far as the cortex. It is an excellent example of the importance of place coding. Tonotopic organization means that information about the place of stimulation is preserved anatomically within the nervous system from the basilar membrane to the cortex.

Some cells in the auditory cortex maintain their firing rate during stimulation, whereas others are affected only at onset or offset. The findings suggest that there may be a sustained–transient, or X–Y division, for audition as there is in vision (see 5.13).

A recent development has come from relating the tonal response of single neurons to the way they respond to speech or other natural sounds. Kiang and Moxon have demonstrated that cat primary auditory neurons, which prefer high frequencies, also play an important role in signalling information about low frequencies at more intense (more normal) levels.

This information has helped resolve a paradox in human hearing. Exposure to intense noise damages hair cells close to the stapes, those hair cells stimulated most by high frequency tones above 5000 Hz. The paradox is that such people have difficulty understanding speech, particularly in noisy environments, even though the main components of speech have a lower frequency (100–5000 Hz) and might be expected to stimulate a relatively undamaged region of the basilar membrane. Kiang and Moxon showed that, although hair cells close to the stapes are tuned to high frequencies, they also respond to speech at normal listening levels. If these cells are lost the listener loses one important source of information, resulting in a decrease in intelligibility.

5.21 The vestibular system

The components of the vestibular system in the inner ear act to maintain a stable image on the retina during head movements.

In order to see properly, the visual image must be held fairly stable on the retina. Maintenance of a relatively stable image is not a simple process. As we walk, our heads move. If we move a TV camera the way our heads move during walking, the result is a smeared, jerky sequence of images. Why does this jerky movement not occur under our normal viewing conditions? The answer is that we have sophisticated sensors in our skulls, which respond to head movements and act on the neck muscles to reduce the head movement, and on the eye muscles to rotate the eye to keep the image fairly stationary. The sensors are the components of the vestibular system.

Let us consider another simple demonstration of the importance of vestibular control of eye movements. Move your hand from side to side in front of you, about 4 or 5 times a second, and try to follow your fingers voluntarily. It is difficult, if not impossible, and you experience a smeary blur. If you hold your hand still and move your head from side to side, at 4 or 5 times a second, while fixating your fingers, you will observe a clear image of your fingers. In the latter case your vestibular system was automatically compensating for your head movement, whereas in the former case your eyes were being controlled voluntarily. Clearly, voluntary control of eye movements is inadequate to maintain the clear visual image. This is done automatically by the vestibular system.

Deep in the bones on each side of the head are two symmetrical systems of fluid-filled tubes and sacs. They are the inner ears. The three fluid-filled tubes are called *semicircular canals*. Each tube lies in its own plane and is perpendicular to the other two tubes. In the human the diameter of each semicircle is about 6 mm. Each semicircular canal opens into a fluid-filled sac called the *utricle*, and just below this is another sac called the *saccule*. At one end each tube widens out into a flask-shaped swelling called the *ampulla*, and inside it is a little structure like a hairy saddle called the *crista*. Hair cells on the crista are embedded in a jelly-like material called the *cupula* which seals off the canal. The schematic diagram shows an ampulla opened to reveal the crista and cupula. Each canal is built like this: a semicircular tube, widening at one end housing the crista with the hairs embedded in a jelly-like cupula which seals the tube of the canal. The rest of the circle of fluid is completed in the utricle.

Each of the six canals (three on each side of the head) functions in a similar way. Angular accelerations of the head (turning movements) cause the fluid in the tube to be "left behind" so that it moves within the tube and exerts force on the jelly-like cupula sealing off the tube. This is only a tiny force, but the cupula is extremely flexible so that it is easily displaced and the receptor hair cells in the cupula will be bent. When the hair cells are bent, their resting potential changes, which in turn affects the firing rate of the afferent neurons synapsing with the hair cell, thus signalling that an angular acceleration of the head has occurred.

If the plane of head rotation is the same as the plane of one canal, only the receptors in that canal will be activated. If the plane of head rotation is somewhere between the planes of two

The vestibular system in each inner ear is composed of three tubes (the semicircular canals) and two sacs (the utricle and the saccule). Head acceleration causes receptor hair cells to be bent. The semicircular canals respond to angular acceleration (turning movements). The utricle and saccule respond to linear accelerations (such as gravity).

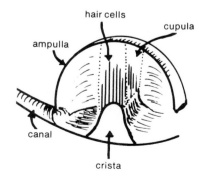

The contents of an ampulla of a semicircular canal.

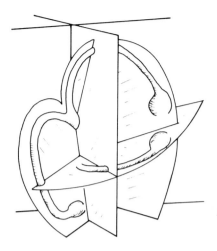

The planes of the semicircular canals in each labyrinth are almost at right angles to each other.

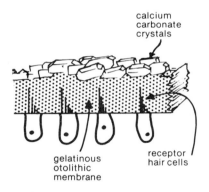

calcium carbonate crystals

gelatinous otolithic membrane

receptor hair cells

Receptor cells of the utricle and saccule.

canals, then the receptors in each canal will be activated. The relative amount of activation depends on how close the plane of head rotation is to the plane of the canal. In most planes of head rotation, all three canals will be activated. The three canals allow a unique pattern of neural input to the brain for each plane of head rotation, just as the three cone types in the retina allow a unique pattern of neural input for each wavelength of light (see 5.8).

The receptor cells in the utricle and saccule are arranged differently, but they work in a similar way to those in the semicircular canals. In each structure there is a fairly flat sheet of tissue with hair cells projecting from it into a gelatinous mass called the *otolithic membrane*. In both the utricle and saccule the membrane is covered with a layer of dense crystals of calcium carbonate. The otolithic membrane can slide over the hair cells and bend them. If the head is tilted or given a linear acceleration, the force acts on the dense otolithic membrane, dragging it in relation to the hair cells, thus bending the hair cells and causing their resting potential to change. The orientation of the flat membranes and the receptor hair cells in the utricle and saccule is such that any possible head tilt can be signalled.

There is an additional complication in the vestibular system. For each canal there is a parallel canal on the other side of the head. When you turn your head, you are stimulating the parallel horizontal canals on both sides of the head. The neural input from a canal on one side of the head interacts with the neural input from its parallel canal on the other side. The neural interaction enhances the sensitivity of the semicircular canal response to angular acceleration.

If you turn your head while fixating a point directly in front of you, your eye will not move with your head. In many situations, voluntary control of eye movements is not efficient enough to explain this simple ability. Rather, as you start to turn your head, the semicircular canal closest to the plane of rotation is activated and neurons from that canal send information along a short, fast neural path to the appropriate eye muscles. The impulses cause the eye muscle to drag on the eyeball in the correct plane to compensate for the movement of the skull. Your eye effectively stays fixed while your head moves, and the image on the retina is not smeared during the head movement.

5.22 Introduction to the skin senses, taste and smell

It may seem odd to group these diverse sensory systems together, but approaches to their study have been similar. The success of an analysis in terms of primary colours in explaining colour vision has led to similar approaches in other sensory modalities. For example, it would be convenient to be able to reduce the enormous variety of smells we experience to a small number of primary smells. Similar attempts have occurred in taste and skin senses. This "primary" approach continues to dominate research on these senses.

5.23 Skin senses

Von Frey argued for four primary skin sensations: touch, heat, cold and pain. He believed that every other skin sensation consisted of combinations of the primary sensations. For example, the sensation of wetness = touch + cold; oiliness = touch + warm. Von Frey proposed a different type of receptor for each primary sensation. Part of the reason for this proposal is that the skin is not uniformly sensitive to each primary. For example, some spots are more sensitive to cold than others. This is easy to demonstrate by the systematic exploration of small patches of skin with a cold probe. The cold is felt at low intensities in some areas, but only at much higher intensities in other areas.

Von Frey postulated that the four primary skin sensations are touch, heat, cold and pain.

Once it had been confirmed that the skin is not uniformly sensitive to the primary sensations, it should have been easy to test Von Frey's proposition. All one had to do was find out how some spot responded (for example, whether it was sensitive to cold) and then cut out that piece of skin and find out what type of receptor lay underneath. Unfortunately that approach does not work. Some cold spots have one type of receptor beneath the skin, other cold spot have other types of receptors. The cornea has only free nerve endings, but displays all the primary sensations although, according to von Frey, free nerve endings were associated specifically with pain. Part of the problem lies in the great variety of receptor types in the skin. There are at least 100 different types, and some are very difficult to distinguish.

An entirely different approach involves recording from a neuron leading to some unknown receptor and examining the stimuli affecting the firing rate of the neuron. The most usual finding is that the firing rate of the neuron can be affected by two or more primary stimuli, such as touch and heat. In other words, neurons conveying the sensory information are non-specific.

Many neurons that convey somatosensory information are not specific to one sensation.

So far, attempts to account for skin sensations in terms of primaries have not been very successful. However, it appears that some receptors and nerve fibres are differentially sensitive; that is, they respond more readily to some kinds of stimuli than to others.

Neural information about some somatosensory stimulation is sent to the brain using a receptive field organization resembling that seen in the visual system. For example, a single neuron can

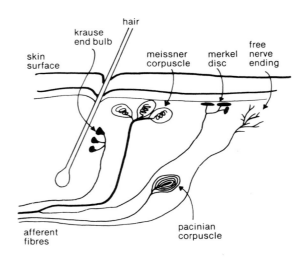

A cross-section through skin showing some of the common receptor types.

be excited by touch in a restricted region of the skin, whereas touching adjacent skin areas causes inhibition. Again, as is the case with vision, there is overlap of the receptive fields, which also vary in size. A further similarity with complex orientation detectors in the visual system is that some somatosensory cortical neurons appear to respond to brushing the skin in one direction but not in the reverse direction.

5.24 Kinaesthesis

Kinaesthesis is the sense of limb position.

Much is known about the sense of limb position, or kinaesthesis. It is perhaps a mistake to discuss kinaesthesis as a sense. It is more like the vestibular system through which our brain is constantly receiving information of which we are usually unaware. We can touch the tip of our noses with our eyes shut fairly easily, but how do we do it? It is really a complex manoeuvre. We must have information about the relative position of our nose, hand and arm, and how fast they are moving. Receptors in the joints signal joint position and velocity of movement, and receptors in the muscles signal information about stretch. All these cues are automatically integrated to allow the performance of nose touching. The study of kinaesthesis has progressed far, perhaps because it has not been burdened with the concept of primaries.

5.25 Pain

All of the other senses are based upon converting a particular form of environmental energy (light, sound, pressure, etc.) into electrochemical information that can be used by he nervous system. Pain is a unique sense in that it is not associated with a single class of stimuli. For example, whereas vision is normally only produced by light, pain may be produced by heat, cold, touch or chemical means. Although these different types of pain do have certain things in common, they also have important differences.

Pain is also unique in that it is the only sense that has a major emotional component. The sensory and emotional aspects of pain can be dissociated by certain drugs. For example, high doses of anti-anxiety agents such as certain tranquilizers do not seriously impair discrimination between stimuli ranging from painless to extremely painful. However, even though subjects may report certain stimuli as being excruciatingly painful they do not seem to care. The drug appears to leave the sensory aspects of pain intact, while almost completely suppressing the emotional aspects. Traditional pain-killers like morphine suppress the sensation of pain itself.

As is the case with the other skin senses, the receptors for pain are not well differentiated structurally. However, it does appear that the major pain receptors are the free nerve endings. The problem is that not all free nerve endings respond to painful stimuli and that many pain-responsive nerve endings also respond to quite different stimuli.

Pain-responsive nerves have been classified on the basis of their fibre diameter as being either large or small. The Gate Control Theory of pain states that pain depends on the relative activity in these two sets of fibres. Pain is associated with one of these sets of fibres being disproportionately activated. This theory is supported by clinical observations that chronic pain may be reduced by electrical stimulation of large diameter fibres. A similar mechanism could underly the analgesia (pain reduction) produced by rubbing a sore spot, or even perhaps the apparent analgesia that may be produced by acupuncture. It should be added that there are also clinical reports where large fibre stimulation has failed to produce analgesia.

Among the most provocative of the recent findings on pain is the demonstration that analgesia can be produced by electrical stimulation of certain sites in the brain stem. Brief periods of brain stimulation can produce long lasting and large magnitude analgesia. The effective sites, which are primarily located near the ventricles, include the periaqueductal grey and raphe magnus. Stimulation-produced analgesia has some parallels with the analgesia produced by morphine, suggesting that there may be a common mode of action of these two analgesic treatments.

Recent discoveries have suggested that the common mode of action of stimulation-produced analgesia and morphine may be due to a common effect on a group of chemical agents in the

There seem to be naturally occurring pain-killers in the brain.

brain called *endorphins*. This term is an abbreviation of "endo-genous morphine-related compounds". The endorphins are naturally occurring compounds composed of chains of amino acids (peptides). A sub-group of these opiate peptides consists of compounds with very few amino acids in the chain, and these short chain compounds have been named enkephalins. There is great hope that these compounds hold the secret to the useful analgesic and the dangerous addictive properties of morphine and related opiate compounds. Enkephalin research is one of the great growth areas of the contemporary neurosciences.

5.26 Taste

The four primary tastes have been held to be salty, sweet, sour and bitter.

Problems arise from attempts to identify primaries for both taste and smell. In taste, the four primaries are held to be salty, sweet, sour and bitter. Again it has been maintained that all tastes can be reduced to combinations of these four primary tastes. As with the skin senses, early research showed that the tongue is not uniformly sensitive to the primary tastes, with the tip being most sensitive to sweet, the sides to sour, and the back to bitter. However, most of the tongue is uniformly sensitive to salt.

On the tongue there are thousands of little mounds of skin. Each mound is called a *papilla*. In some papillae the taste receptor cells are grouped together to form *taste buds*. There are about five taste buds per papilla, and in each bud about 40–60 receptor cells are arranged like segments in an orange. Each taste receptor has little hairs at the top and the hairs project into a small crater in the papilla. It is thought that taste reception occurs at these hairs.

Pfaffman examined the responses of single taste nerve fibres to various solutions in a number of species, including man. Typically, the firing rate of a fibre is increased by different solutions.

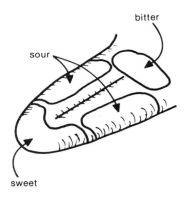

Different parts of the tongue are most sensitive to three of the primary tastes.

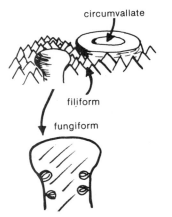

A small area of tongue showing three different types of papilla.

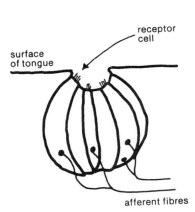

The cells of one taste bud.

Each fibre seems to be more sensitive to some solutions than to others, but there is none of the specificity required by a "primary" account of tastes. For example, one fibre may be excited by both salt and saccharin. Pfaffman has developed a pattern theory of taste which attributes taste quality to the relative amount of activity in all afferent neurons from the tongue. Again, the idea of primaries has not been successful.

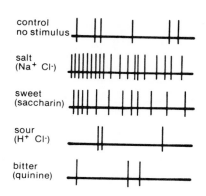

A single neuron from the tongue can be excited by different primary tastes.

5.27 Smell

The limited amount of research carried out on smell indicates a non-specificity similar to that found in taste. Even so, there have been attempts to reduce all smells to seven primaries. In a recent study, Amoore considered how chemists describe the smell of compounds and identified seven primary odours: camphoraceous, musky, floral, ethereal, minty, pungent, and putrid. However, this system has met with little more success than the primary systems in other modalities.

The receptors for smell are hair cells situated in a recess in the nasal cavity. The hairs project into a mucus layer and molecules of the odorous substance must dissolve in this mucus to reach the receptor hair cells. Recordings of neural activity from fibres synapsing with these receptor cells have again shown non-specificity. Some fibres respond to many "primary" smells, but are more sensitive to some than to others.

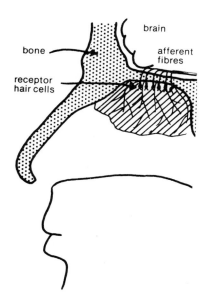

The striped area shows the location of the receptor cells for smell.

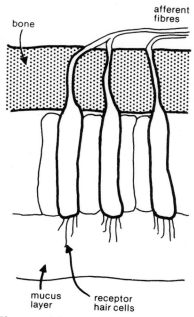

Close-up of the receptor cells for smell.

camphoraceous   floral

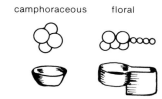

Amoore has hypothesized that the different primary odours have different shaped molecules which fit exactly into appropriately shaped recesses in the membrane of the receptor cells, triggering changes in neural activity.

Amoore has developed a "lock and key" theory of smell based on the molecular shapes of substances corresponding to the seven primary odours. The molecular models of the substances Amoore studied suggested to him that there is a distinct molecular size or shape corresponding to each odour primary. He hypothesized that each receptor contains a recess of a size and shape adapted to that of the molecule to which it is tuned. When a molecule of appropriate size and shape is present, it locks into the recess, and the resting potential of the cell is altered. Primary molecules fit their recesses exactly. Other molecules fit the recesses of a number of primary odours and so produce a combination of primaries resulting in the distinct quality of many odours.

Amoore's theory has had a novel test. He has been able to synthesize completely novel compounds with a particular molecular size and shape and predict how they should smell, in some cases with considerable success. Unfortunately certain compounds smell alike, although their molecular structures are different. On the other hand some compounds smell different although their molecular structures are similar. His current research is directed at identifying individuals who are "smell-blind"; that is, they are insensitive to some odours, just as colour-blind people are insensitive to certain colours. Colour blindess has provided important evidence for the concept of primary colours. Amoore maintains that smell-blindness may lead to a similar confirmation of the concept of odour primaries.

5.28 Conclusion

In the skin senses, in taste and in smell, the analysis of stimulation in terms of primaries has met with little success. In each of these senses recordings from afferent fibres have shown a considerable degree of non-specificity. One suggestion is that the non-specificity may be caused by the high concentrations or intensities of the stimuli used. For example, if high intensity tones are used to study the responses of a single auditory neuron, then the neuron will respond to a range of frequencies. However, as the intensity of the tones is reduced, the neuron's response becomes more and more specific. At very low intensities the neuron will respond to only one frequency. By analogy, Von Békésy suggested that possibly the intensities used in studying taste may have been too high so that the taste neurons respond to a range of tastes. He reported that, when very low intensity taste stimuli were used, there was specificity. However, others have not been able to repeat his observations. Thus, it remains to be seen whether analysing these sensory systems in terms of primaries is the appropriate research strategy.

Questions

General principles of coding

1 Do our senses faithfully tell us about the physical world? Give examples.
2 What is adaptation?
3 To what principle does the occurrence of adaptation seem to point?
4 How can the brain discriminate between senses?
5 What is Müller's doctrine? What problems does it encounter?
6 Generally, what effects does increasing stimulus intensity have?
7 What is inhibition? Why is it important in neural coding?
8 What is unusual about the coding of adjacent stimuli?

Vision

9 What is the range of wavelengths of visible light?
10 What happens to white light when passed through a prism?
11 What colour results when all visible wavelengths are added together?
12 Where is the cornea?
13 Where is the pupil?
14 What is the iris?
15 What is the retina?
16 Why do the eyes of some animals shine in the dark?
17 What are you looking at when you look at someone's pupil?
18 Explain how the iris works.
19 What structures bring the image to a focus on the retina?
20 What is accommodation?
21 Why do old people hold newspapers at arms' length to read them?
22 How is the retina connected to the brain?
23 Objects in the left half of your visual field project to which half of the brain?
24 Name the photoreceptors and their relative numbers.
25 On what part of the retina is the density of cones greatest?
26 On what part of the retina is the density of rods greatest?
27 What is the optic disc and why is it significant?
28 At what average light levels do the two retinal systems function?
29 Why is there a kink in the curve for recovery from light adaptation?
30 If someone without cones were tested for recovery from light adaptation what should the results look like?
31 What is a quantum?
32 How are the rod and cone systems "hooked up" to retinal ganglion cells?
33 Why do objects look grey at low light levels?
34 What is colour?
35 To what wavelength is the rod system most sensitive?
36 What is the Purkinje shift?
37 Why do rods not permit colour vision?
38 How do cones permit colour vision?
39 What is the Young–Helmholtz Trichromatic Theory of colour vision?
40 How can additive colour mixture be explained?
41 How can colour blindness be explained?
42 What are complementary colours?

43 What is Hering's theory of colour vision?
44 What is a negative after-image?
45 What did De Valois discover about the neural coding of wavelength?
46 What is a contour?
47 What is lateral inhibition and what is its apparent function?
48 What are Mach bands and how is lateral inhibition consistent with them?
49 Explain how human perceptual phenomena can be consistent with lateral inhibition.
50 What is a receptive field?
51 What are the characteristics of receptive fields of retinal ganglion cells?
52 How can it be shown that ON and OFF regions are mutually antagonistic?
53 What is a spatial summation in a retinal ganglion cell?
54 Why are retinal ganglion cells sometimes called edge detectors?
55 How does antagonism between ON and OFF regions permit the visual system to function over a large range of intensities?
56 Describe the typical receptive fields of simple visual cortical cells.
57 Why have such cells been called orientation detectors?
58 What are the characteristics of complex and hypercomplex cells?
59 What is the hierarchical theory?
60 Why is it not complete?
61 Approximately how many visual cortical cells are binocular?
62 What are the structural correlates of orientation in the visual cortex?
63 What are the W, X, Y systems and why are they so named?
64 Describe the characteristics of Y-type retinal ganglion cells.
65 To where do they project?
66 Describe the characteristics of the X-type retinal ganglion cells.
67 What is one suggested function of W cells?
68 What is a plausible account of the function of the X and Y systems?
69 How does early visual experience affect a cat's visual cortical cells?
70 What is the critical period?
71 What is astigmatism and why has it been important in studies of the development of vision?

Hearing
72 What is sound?
73 What is the frequency of a tone?
74 What is the amplitude of a tone?
75 What are pitch and loudness?
76 What is psychophysics?
77 What are the limits of hearing of young adults?
78 Which part of the inner ear is concerned with hearing?
79 Describe the anatomy of the cochlea.
80 How do sounds reach it?
81 What is the basilar membrane and why is it important?
82 Describe events in the inner ear during stimulation by a pure tone.
83 Where do low frequency pure tones cause maximum basilar membrane displacement? And high frequencies?
84 How does decreasing the amplitude of a low frequency tone affect the pattern of basilar membrane displacement?
85 What is a tuning curve?

86   Why does your voice sound thin when you hear it replayed by a tape recorder?
87   What is conductive deafness? Can it be treated?
88   In what sense is the neural coding of frequency determined in multiple ways?
89   Why has sharpening been suggested in hearing?
90   What are the characteristics of neural coding in the auditory cortex?
91   Why do people with damage to the high frequency region of the basilar membrane have trouble understanding the predominantly low frequency stimulus of speech?

Vestibular system
92   What function does the vestibular system serve?
93   What are the anatomical structures making up the vestibular system?
94   Which part is stimulated by angular acceleration and how does it occur?
95   If one of the two vestibular systems in your head were damaged what consequences would you expect?
96   What are the suggested primary skin sensations?
97   Name two problems with the "primary" approach to skin sensations?
98   What is kinesthesis and what permits it?
99   What do acupuncture and opium have in common neurally?
100 What are the suggested primary tastes?
101 What is a taste bud?
102 What do we mean when we say that taste nerve fibres are non-specific?
103 What are the suggested primary smells?
104 What is Amoore's theory of smell and how has he tested it?
105 Why might stimulus intensity be important in tests of primaries in the various senses?

Further Readings

Frisby, J.P. *Seeing: Illusion, Brain and Mind.* Oxford, Oxford University Press. 1979.
Hubel, D.H. and Wiesel, T.N. Brain mechanisms of vision. *Scientific American,* 1979, **241** (3), 130–144.
Ludel, J. *Introduction to Sensory Processes.* San Francisco, Ca., W.H. Freeman. 1978.
Moore, B.C.J. *Hearing.* London, Macmillan. 1977.

6

Sleep and Wakefulness

6.1 Biological rhythms

Many aspects of our behaviour and physiology change with a strikingly regular pattern. Some of these rhythmic changes are obviously responses to certain environmental demands. For example, our daytime behaviour is quite different from our night-time behaviour because daytime is typically a time of work and activity. However other behaviours appear to be triggered by internal processes. These internally generated patterns of behavioural and physiological changes are called *biological rhythms*. Perhaps the most obvious biological rhythm is our daily cycle of sleep and wakefulness. The cycle has a time period of about 24 hours and is consequently called a *circadian rhythm* (from the Latin meaning about one day). Animals with circadian sleep–wakefulness cycles may be either *diurnal* (day active) *nocturnal* (night active) or, as is common in birds, *crepuscular* (dawn and dusk active). Whereas these cycles have an obvious relationship to environmental changes such as sunrise and sunset, considerations presented below suggest that to a large extent they are internally generated.

Biological rhythms are found in nearly all behavioural and physiological systems.

Although circadian rhythms are the best known biological rhythms, there are other rhythms with different time periods. Biological rhythms with a time period of less than 24 hours are called *ultradian rhythms*. Examples of biological rhythms with a time period greater than 24 hours are the *circumlunar* (approximately one month) female menstruation cycles and the *circannial* (approximately one year) cycles of breeding and migration seen in many animals.

Biological rhythms affect virtually every physiological and

biochemical process in the body as well as many behavioural responses. Body temperature, urine production and energy utilization all have circadian rhythms. Some people are clearly "night-owls" who function best after sundown. Other people are "early-birds" who function best during the day. Experiments have shown that the resistance to the stress of oxygen deprivation may be as much as 50% greater at certain times of the day. It is likely that the resistance to other stressors may also vary with a circadian rhythm. Pain sensitivity and the analgesic effect of drugs vary greatly over the day. In fact, it appears that the effects of many drugs may be quite different at different times of the day. Since the rhythms of the effects and side effects may peak at different times of the day, it may be possible to temporally "tailor" drug dosages to maximize the desired therapeutic affects and to minimize undesirable side effects. Conversely, depending on drug-effect relationships with the relevant biological rhythms, a given drug dose could at different times of the day be an ineffective underdose or a potentially lethal overdose.

The effects of drugs vary markedly at different times of the day.

The independence of biological rhythms from environmental cues suggests that the rhythms may be generated by what is commonly referred to as a biological clock. The existence of a biological clock is suggested by the persistence of biological rhythms when environmental cues are eliminated. For example, under conditions of continuous light or darkness, rhythms of sleep–wakefulness, body temperature and hormonal secretions continue for long periods of time.

The persistence of biological rhythms when external cues are removed or altered suggests that they are generated by an internal biological clock.

The various biological rhythms peak at different times, and there are large individual differences in the patterning of these peaks. Since the period of diurnal rhythms is rarely exactly 24 hours, there is a tendency for them to drift. However, it appears that cues of light and dark "re-set" most of the rhythms each day, thus preventing drift and keeping the rhythms in a fixed temporal relationship with day and night. If this temporal relationship is suddenly altered by a long intercontinental flight, a disconcerting and disrupting situation called "jet lag" is produced. Since the rhythms can only be reset gradually, it may take days to recover from jet lag.

Diurnal rhythms have a period of about 24 hours.

6.2 Defining sleep

The sleep–wakefulness cycle is the most obvious biological rhythm. Unlike other biological rhythms which are quantitative fluctuations about some mean value, the sleep–wakefulness cycle represents a qualitative shift between fundamentally different states of consciousness.

Defining sleep is rather more difficult than it may at first seem. The "waking" state can reasonably be defined as the absence of sleeping. This, of course, necessitates an adequate definition of sleep. Sleep has traditionally been defined by the occurrence of recumbent posture, eye closure, muscle relaxation, reduced autonomic activity and reduced reactivity to environmental stimuli. Since all of these changes can also occur during the relaxed waking state, there is an obvious need for unequivocal indicators of sleep. We will see below that sleep may be defined by a number of distinct electrophysiological characteristics.

In 1929, Berger made an historic breakthrough which led to an electrophysiological definition of sleep. Berger noticed that he could record very small and rapidly fluctuating electrical potentials from the head of his infant son. He correctly presumed that these voltage changes, which are called the *electroencephalogram* (EEG), reflected the electrical activity of the brain. The EEG varied according to the child's state of alertness.

Sleep may be defined by characteristic changes in the electroencephalogram (EEG).

Special patterns of EEG activity, as well as the electrical activity of certain muscle groups, can reliably differentiate sleep from wakefulness. Rather surprisingly, it was later found that these same indicators allowed the differentiation of two fundamentally different states of sleep (see 6.4). Thus electrophysiological research has identified three quite distinct states of consciousness. The two states of consciousness collectively covered by the term "sleep" are most commonly known as *slow-wave sleep* and *rapid eye-movement sleep*.

There are two distinct states of sleep — slow-wave sleep and rapid eye-movement (REM) sleep.

6.3 Slow-wave sleep

During the waking state the EEG contains large amounts of very high-frequency, low-amplitude activity. This is referred to as the *beta-rhythm*. As we relax and close our eyes, the EEG begins to show low-frequency (8–12 Hz) and higher-amplitude activity which is called the *alpha-rhythm*. The transition to sleep is marked by an increase in the alpha content of the EEG plus the appearance of the even lower-frequency (1–4 Hz) and higher-amplitude *delta-rhythm*. This slowing and regularization of the EEG is referred to as *synchronization*. Because of this characteristic EEG activity, this state of sleep is referred to as slow-wave sleep. It is also sometimes called delta or synchronized sleep.

Slow-wave sleep is characterized by a gradual slowing and synchronization of the EEG.

As the electrical activity of the brain becomes synchronized during sleep, there are also general reductions in the activity of both striped (skeletal) and smooth (autonomic) muscle. These muscular changes reduce eye movements and blood pressure as well as heart and respiration rates. The reductions in the activity of the brain and muscles are accompanied by reduced responsiveness to environmental stimuli. It appears that during slow-wave sleep the organism is generally winding down or "running out of steam". These data have been used to support the notion that sleep is simply a passive lapse out of wakefulness. However, even within the state of slow-wave sleep there are some phenomena which suggest that sleep is an active phenomena. We do not simply fall out of wakefulness, rather we actively fall into sleep.

Sleep is an active phenomenon. It is not simply a passive lapse out of wakefulness.

Besides numerous suggestions from the neural mechanisms of sleep (see 6.8), an active theory of slow-wave sleep is supported by the changes in pupil size and reactivity to environmental stimuli that occur during slow-wave sleep. The pupils become smaller — an active muscle response. Someone who is not awake and still shows a large pupil opening is very likely to be dead. The generally reduced responsiveness to environmental stimulation occurs while some sensory "channels" apparently remain wide open. For example, a mother may well sleep through loud traffic noises but will quickly awake to the slightest sound from her child. It appears that we no more passively fall out of waking into sleep than we fall out of sleep into waking. Each of these states of consciousness has active neural mechanisms for their initiation, maintenance and termination.

6.4 Rapid eye-movement sleep

The overall sleep cycle of humans, in particular, consists of two quite distinct cycles which alternate throughout the night. At about 90 minute intervals slow-wave sleep is replaced by about 15 minute intervals of rapid eye-movement (REM) sleep. Thus the two sleep states are ultradian rhythms within the circadian rhythm of sleep–wakefulness.

REM sleep and slow-wave sleep alternate cyclically throughout the night.

REM sleep appears to be a very deep sleep as judged by an extreme lack of responsiveness to external stimulation, the almost complete abolition of resting muscle tone and greatly reduced autonomic activity. These findings are consistent with the view that REM sleep is simply a deeper stage of slow-wave sleep. However, a number of other features of REM sleep are so completely different from those of slow-wave sleep that REM sleep is now generally agreed to be a qualitatively different *state* — a third state of consciousness.

One of the most remarkable features of REM sleep is that, although some indicators suggest a very deep state of sleep, the EEG is like that of someone who is awake and alert. This peculiar pattern of intense cortical activation during sleep has led to REM sleep also being called *paradoxical* or *activated* sleep.

Muscle activity during REM sleep is also unusual. While autonomic and skeletal activity is generally at a very low level, there are occasional flurries of intense activity. Thus, during REM sleep the generally very low heart rate, blood pressure and respiration rate will occasionally show large increases. Similarly,

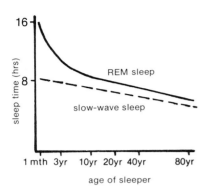

The decline of REM sleep in humans with increasing age.

REM sleep may be an internally programmed stimulation mechanism of particular importance during early infancy.

Sleep disorders are far more common than most people realize.

the almost total lack of skeletal activity will occasionally be interrupted by jerky limb movements. The eyes, which are almost completely immobile during slow-wave sleep, show occasional bursts of movement that are actually more rapid than those seen during waking. It is this pattern of vigorous eye movements that gave this state of sleep its most common name – REM sleep.

REM sleep is found in widely varying degrees in all mammals. Cats spend much of their sleep time in REM sleep, whereas chickens show very little REM sleep. In all species there is a large decline in REM sleep with age. Newborn human infants spend most of their time sleeping, and of this time over 80% is REM sleep. In contrast, adults spend about 15–20% of their sleep cycle in REM sleep.

Roffwarg has developed an intriguing hypothesis to account for the large decline in REM sleep with age. His hypothesis is based on a large body of data which show that environmental stimulation enhances the development of infants (see Ch.10). However, the infant has little muscular ability and cultural habits usually confine infants to a minimally stimulating environment. Thus, just when infants most need stimulation, physiological and cultural limitations prevent them from getting it. Roffwarg argues that REM sleep is a form of internally programmed stimulation which counteracts the sensory deprivation of infancy.

Quite apart from its numerous unusual features there is considerable interest in REM sleep because of its association with dreaming (see 6.6).

6.5 Sleep disorders

A rather surprising by-product of sleep research is the discovery that a great many people suffer from sleep disorders. Approximately one-third of the population report that they sleep too much, too little, fitfully or at inappropriate times.

The most common sleep disorder is *insomnia*, which is characterized by daytime sleepiness which the patients attribute to the inability to sleep at night. Even though insomniacs say that they do not sleep well or enough at night, independent monitoring of their sleep sometimes shows that their night sleep is, in fact, quite normal. This latter condition of daytime sleepiness in spite of normal nightime sleep is more properly called *hypersomnia*.

The traditional treatment for insomnia has been sleeping pills. Although sleeping pills induce sleep, there is a rapid development of tolerance to their effects. This tolerance necessitates increasing doses, which increases their addictive potential. In addition, withdrawal from sleeping pills often results in a long period of unusually poor sleep that is frequently accompanied by nightmares. Thus, in many cases, sleeping pills constitute another example of the treatment being worse than the disease.

Sleeping pills are at best a short-term solution to insomnia.

As pointed out in sections 6.3 and 6.4, sleep is generally characterized as a period of skeletal inactivity. The main exception to this inactivity is the periodic activity seen in REM sleep. A less well-known exception is the fact that most people apparently at some time or other talk in their sleep. Sleep-talking has no particular association with REM sleep and has not been associated with any psychological disturbances. In fact, very little is known about either sleep-talking or the far less common phenomenon of sleep-walking.

Since sleep-talking and sleep-walking suggest that we have hidden motor abilities while sleeping, there has been speculation that we may also retain intellectual abilities during sleep. This belief generated a very substantial business in devices to aid sleep-learning. The notion of effortless learning during what would otherwise be lost time has considerable appeal. There is, unfortunately, no evidence that a significant amount of learning does take place during sleep. If anything, the data suggest a certain amount of amnesia for what occurs during sleep. This is why dreams are difficult to recall and why sleep-talkers and sleep-walkers rarely remember their unusual behaviour. Thus sleep-learning appears to be a dead issue, a curiosity of the 1960s.

Very little, if any, learning appears to take place during sleep.

Another sleep disorder called *sleep apnea* is simply an exaggeration of the reduction in respiratory rate that occurs during sleep. In some unfortunate individuals, the respiratory rate during sleep may be too low to adequately oxygenate the blood. As a result, these people wake up gasping for air. Since sleeping pills also tend to decrease respiratory rate, they are a particularly dangerous and inappropriate medication for sleep apnea. The cot-death syndrome seen in infants may be a manifestation of sleep apnea at a stage before the life-saving gasping reflex has developed.

One of the most serious sleep disorders is *narcolepsy*. Although narcolepsy has a number of distinct symptoms, it may best be described as a sleep attack. The narcoleptic is suddenly and almost without warning plunged into deep (usually REM) sleep. These sleep attacks may be occasional and disturbing or frequent in which case they are severely debilitating. Some narcoleptics are almost totally incapacitated and quite incapable of being gainfully employed. The most common treatment for narcolepsy is the prescription of stimulant drugs such as amphetamines. However, much as is the case with sleeping pills, there is a rapid development of tolerance and addiction to amphetamines. Further, amphetamines may induce psychotic breakdowns (see 11.5).

Narcolepsy may be described as a sudden sleep attack.

6.6 Dreaming

Dreaming is one of the most dramatic and puzzling aspects of sleep. For thousands of years, mystics, prophets and ordinary people have been fascinated by the meaning of these nocturnal adventures. The meaning of dreams has figured very prominently in psychoanalytic theories. However, since dream content is usually interpreted as being highly symbolic, and the interpretation of the symbols is completely subjective, it is not surprising that the psychoanalytic approach has not been very fruitful. It would be quite likely that ten different psychoanalysts would interpret the same dream ten different ways.

The meaning of dreams has also been experimentally investigated by manipulating various aspects of everyday life and then examining subsequent dream content. Sexual stimulation tends to increase the sexual content of dreams, whereas physical exercise tends to decrease the exercise content of dreaming. It is interesting to note that the most common dream content is physical activity, whereas the proportion of sexual content is usually very small. It is also noteworthy that all people dream, although some people do not remember their dreams. This can be shown by simple training procedures which allow even sworn non-dreamers to recall their dreams.

It is generally accepted that REM sleep is the time during which we are most likely to dream. If people are awakened from REM sleep, 80% of the time they will report that they have been dreaming. In contrast, if people are awakened from slow-wave sleep, they will report dreams only about 20% of the time. These findings have led to the speculation that since dreams have abundant visual imagery, perhaps the eye movements represent the "acting out" of visual experiences. However, REMs occur in people who have been blind from birth.

6.7 The function of sleep

It seems eminently reasonable that sleep serves some biological function. Sleep is widely viewed as a period of repair and restoration of the physiological wear and tear that occurs during waking activity. If there is a need for sleep, then sleep should share some common features with other biological needs such as eating. The need for eating is suggested by its occurrence in all species. More direct evidence for the need to eat is provided by examining the effects of preventing eating. Food deprivation produces a striking pattern of changes that will ultimately result in death.

In contrast with other biological needs, sleep does not occur in all species. Some species such as the tree sloth may spend 80%

The interpretation of the meaning of dreams has seen little progress during the past several thousand years.

Everyone appears to dream, although some people have difficulty in recalling their dreams.

Dreams are most likely to occur during REM sleep.

All animals eat, drink and breathe, yet many animals do not sleep.

of their lives asleep, whereas chickens show very little sleep at all. These data suggest that if there is a need for sleep, it is a unique need in that it is confined to vertebrates. Further, most species tend to show numerous brief periods of sleep rather than the single long period of sleep seen in humans. In some cases these sleep episodes may only be a few minutes in duration. It is hard to imagine much restoration taking place in such a short period of time. Most simply, there is no direct evidence that any biological restoration does occur even in the long sleep periods of humans.

The most frequently cited data supporting the need for sleep came from a few cases of observing the effects of long periods of sleep deprivation. Sleep deprivation has been reported to produce an array of psychiatric symptoms ranging from mild depression and hostility to vivid hallucinations. However, these dramatic effects may well have been artifactual. In some of these cases the effects of sleep deprivation were confounded with the effects of food deprivation, exercise and the stressors used to keep the subjects awake. In others, the experimenter conveyed to the subjects their expectancies (or hopes) that something dramatic should happen. In these cases it appears that the subjects may well have "played the game".

Human sleep deprivation studies have all too often generated artifactually sensational results.

In more controlled experiments involving larger numbers of subjects, the effects of sleep deprivation are enough to induce a yawn. People who have been deprived of sleep for up to 11 days become irritable, easily distracted and very sleepy. After 9 days of sleep deprivation one subject was consistently beating the experimenters best scores on a pinball machine. These results certainly argue against sleep deprivation producing the dramatic and even disastrous consequences that have occasionally been reported.

Overall these data raise the interesting and heretical possibility that there is no need for sleep — that sleep serves no biological function. The persistence and insistence of sleep could represent a vestigial biological rhythm. At one time earlier in our evolutionary history sleep may have served a restorative function. However, through the course of evolution we gradually became capable of accomplishing the restoration during waking. Sleep may have persisted even though, like our appendix, it no longer served any purpose.

6.8 Brain mechanisms of sleep and wakefulness

The role of the brain in sleep was first explored by damaging various parts of the brain and observing the effects on the sleep–wakefulness cycle. These early experiments implicated certain parts of the brain stem as sleep centres. For example, cutting the anterior brain stem produced an animal that appeared to be permanently asleep. However, cutting the posterior brain stem had little effect on the sleep–wakefulness cycle. These data were interpreted as indicating that wakefulness was maintained by ascending input from the brain stem to the higher (likely cortical) regions of the brain. Thus, in the absence of excitation, the brain was thought to fall asleep. Note that this is a classic example of a passive theory of sleep. The brain stem system that maintains cortical arousal is the *reticular activating system*. This system is a very large and complex group of nuclei and fibre tracts that, in a sense, form the core of the brain stem. As might be expected, electrical stimulation of the reticular activating system was shown to produce both EEG and behavioural signs of arousal.

Whereas a passive brain stem theory of sleep persisted well into the 1950s, later research showed that sleep is neither a passive phenomenon, nor is it under the exclusive control of brain stem structures. The active nature of sleep was demonstrated by the fact that cutting the brain stem at about the mid-level appeared to produce a permanently awake cat. Thus anterior brain stem cuts produced excessive sleep, mid-level cuts produced excessive wakefulness, and posterior cuts had no effect at all. These data suggest that sleep is not simply a passive lapse from wakefulness. Rather, both sleep and wakefulness are actively maintained by discrete areas of the brain stem, and as we will see below, other brain areas as well.

Sleep and wakefulness are actively maintained by discrete areas in the brain stem which also act in conjunction with other brain areas.

A number of experimenters showed that electrical and chemical stimulation of certain parts of the thalamus and hypothalamus could also induce sleep or wakefulness. Perhaps even more important evidence for the role of midbrain and forebrain structures in the sleep–wakefulness cycle comes from an examination of the long-term effects of the anterior brain stem cuts. In these experiments the anterior brain stem cuts produced the expected excessive sleepiness that was evident immediately after the operation. However, about two weeks after the operations the experimental animals began to show a gradual and steady recovery of sleep–wakefulness cycles. Thus it seems that the brain can maintain this fundamental rhythm, even when disconnected from the brain stem sites that were once thought to be sleep–wakefulness "centres". These experiments once again illustrate the point that brain functions are rarely centered. Instead, they are typically represented by systems which may extend over large areas of the brain.

Whereas many different brain manipulations produce short-term alterations in the sleep-wakefulness cycle, long-term changes are very rare.

An equally important implication of these experiments is that the short-term effects of brain lesions may be very different from the long-term effects. Consequently, the many lesion experiments which still focus almost exclusively on short-term effects may provide an incorrect view of the functions subserved by various parts of the brain. This is particularly true when the lesions produce an impairment or a reduction in any function.

Perhaps the dominant theory of the brain mechanisms of sleep has been developed by Jouvet and his colleagues in France. Basically, Jouvet's theory depicts two brain stem sites that are anatomically and neurochemically distinct: one controls slow-wave sleep and the other controls REM sleep. Jouvet observed that damage to the brain stem *raphe complex* produced insomnia. The raphe complex was shown to be the site of origin of many of the forebrain serotonin neurons. Drugs which reduced serotonergic function also produced insomnia. These data formed the core of a raphe–serotonergic theory of slow-wave sleep.

It was also reported that damage to the brain stem *locus coeruleus* eliminated REM sleep. The locus coeruleus was shown to be the site of origin of many of the forebrain noradrenalin neurons. Drugs which reduced noradrenergic function tended to eliminate REM sleep. However, much as was the case with the brain stem cuts which altered the sleep–wakefulness cycle, lesions or changes which affect the raphe complex or the locus coeruleus may only have transient disruptive effects. In spite of large raphe or locus coeruleus lesions, long-term sleep patterns return to normal. Similarly, in long-term amphetamine addicts (who presumably have altered noradrenergic activity) sleep–wakefulness cycles are essentially normal. All of these data suggest that sleep–wakefulness cycles are far more neurochemically complex than was originally believed.

One source of the new-found neurochemical complexity of sleep–wakefulness is the discovery of certain peptides (short chains of amino acids) which can selectively affect various components of the sleep–wakefulness cycle. Although these peptides have not yet been structurally characterized, they hold great promise for clarifying important aspects of this longstanding problem.

Questions

1 Is slow-wave sleep necessary?
2 Is rapid eye-movement sleep necessary?
3 Discuss the therapy of sleep disorders.
4 What are dreams, and what do they signify?

Further Readings

Drucker-Colin, R.R. and Spanis, C.W. Is there a sleep transmitter? *Progress in Neurobiology*, 1976, **6**, 1–22.
Horne, J.A. A review of the biological effects of total sleep deprivation in man. *Biological Psychology*, 1978, **7**, 55–102.

Petre-Quadens, O. and Schlag, J.D. *Basic Sleep Mechanisms*. New York, Academic Press. 1974.
Ramm, P. The locus coeruleus, Catecholamines and REM sleep: A critical review. *Behavioral and Neural Biology*, 1979, **25**, 415–448.

7

Physiological Regulatory Mechanisms

7.1 Introduction

Living organisms are biological machines which, like other machines, have certain physical needs that must be met. Failure to meet these needs in the short term produces functional abnormalities and in the long term death. The complexity of physiological machinery is reflected in the number of factors which must be regulated to ensure optimal functioning. Some of these factors are: energy balance; fluid balance; body temperature; acid–base balance; electrolyte balance; and oxygen levels. This list is by no means complete, and it should be noted that these factors are strongly interdependent. A disruption in any of these regulatory systems inevitably produces disruptions in the others.

Evolution has endowed us with an elaborate set of regulatory mechanisms which serve to maintain the vital physiological factors within a narrow range. When these factors are regulated within the prescribed range, an organism is said to be in a state of equilibrium or homeostasis (from the Greek meaning "same state"). Traditionally, the disruption of physiological homeostasis has been considered to be a cause of various drives and motivation. Although "drive" and "motivation" are terms still used in the life sciences, scepticism about their general usefulness has recently emerged. The problem is that, when behaviour is explained as being the result of drives and motivation, one is still left with the problem of explaining the drives and motivation. In contrast to behavioural terms, drive and motivational terms are not well defined. In fact, motivation is commonly inferred from the very behaviour that it is said to explain. The physiological approach may have a great deal to

The notion of 'set-points' is borrowed from control theory, and in some physiological systems their definition is rather imprecise.

contribute to this long-standing problem by providing an independent way of defining drives and motivation.

The optimal value for any physiological parameter (variable) is sometimes called a *set-point*. The set-points of some parameters, such as body temperature (37°), are easily specified and are essentially invariant within the life-span of an individual or even between species. The set-points of other parameters, such as body weight, are less easily specified since body weight varies considerably even within the life-span of a member of one species. Among members of a species or between different species the variability of body weight becomes enormous. In particular, the variability of body weight has generated considerable reluctance in accepting it as a regulated parameter. Body weight is sometimes seen as the rather incidental outcome of regulating other factors such as food intake. We will see below that there are considerable advantages in considering body weight as a regulated parameter somewhat like body temperature.

7.2 Traditional peripheral theories of body-weight regulation

Early peripheral theories emphasized the importance of local sensations from the mouth and stomach as the cause of eating and drinking.

Because of the obvious association between the stomach and eating, the stomach figured prominently in early theories of body-weight regulation. Stomach distension after a meal may be a signal to finish eating. Conversely, people frequently speak of their stomach "growling" before meals. Such informal observations were formalized in a theory of Cannon and his colleagues earlier this century. They claimed that "hunger nerves" in the stomach were irritated by contractions of an empty stomach. Distension produced by eating was thought to soothe the hunger nerves and produce satiety. Similarly, thirst was attributed to sensations arising from a dry mouth, and satiation of thirst was attributed to a wet mouth.

Peripheral sensory cues may play a role under certain conditions, but there is evidence that their contribution to overall body-weight regulation is slight. For example, recent experiments show that an empty stomach may be inactive and a full stomach active, the reverse of predictions from the original local theories. Furthermore, humans with denervated stomachs or with no stomachs at all, report normal sensations of hunger and can regulate their body-weight as well as people with intact stomachs. Peripheral theories of drinking face the same problems. Removal of the salivary glands results in a dry mouth, yet there is no overall increase in water intake. Similarly, we know that thirst is not relieved by rinsing one's mouth with water. The demise of the early peripheralist theories was not simply due to inconsistent and contrary evidence, but to the development of a theory that accounted more completely for the known facts of body-weight regulation.

7.3 Monitoring of body weight

Evidence shows that the brain plays a major role in body-weight regulation. However, before considering the contribution of various brain nuclei and systems, we shall consider the question of how the brain, as a first step in regulation, senses our body weight.

Most organisms regulate weight in the absence of bathroom scales, indicating an ability to make use of other indirect cues related to body weight.

Body weight is generally monitored indirectly through various cues related to the state of our energy balance.

7.4 Thermostatic monitoring

Since there is evidence that certain cells in the brain are particularly responsive to temperature changes, some investigators have attempted to implicate thermostatic mechanisms in the initiation and termination of eating. Such theories, primarily developed by Brobeck and colleagues, can be summarized as "eat for heat". According to this theory, a food deficit produces a shortage of metabolic fuel, resulting in lower metabolic activity and consequently lower body temperature. The temperature change is detected by hypothalamic cells which then initiate eating. Eating, by supplying metabolic fuel, results in increased metabolic activity and consequently increased temperature. It is thought that the termination of eating is due to the temperature increase.

According to the thermostatic view, the initiation of eating is triggered by low body temperature and the termination of eating is triggered by high body temperature.

The thermostatic theory is supported by observations that food intake tends to increase in a cold environment and decrease in a warm environment. Also, other experiments show that the temperature of the hypothalamus does increase during feeding. However, Grossman has shown that meal size does not correlate with hypothalamic temperature, either at the start or at the end of a meal.

Grossman has obtained even more direct evidence against the theory. The hypothalamus is located directly above the roof of the mouth, and relatively large changes in hypothalamic temperature ($\pm 5°C$) can be brought about simply by eating hot or cold food. If organsims "eat for heat", it would be expected that they need to eat far more cold food than hot food, yet no such differences were found by Grossman. These observations suggest that under normal conditions thermostatic mechanisms play only a minor role in body-weight regulation.

7.5 Glucostatic monitoring

Glucose is an important energy source, particularly for brain metabolism, and is therefore a probable cue to body weight. The glucostatic theory, principally developed by Mayer and colleagues, states in its simplest form that the initiation of eating is associated with low blood glucose levels, whereas the termination of eating is associated with high blood glucose levels. The changes in blood glucose levels are thought to be detected by specialized cells in the hypothalamus called glucoreceptors. Microelectrode recordings confirm the presence of hypothalamic cells that are particularly responsive to glucose.

However, some clinical data from diabetics indicate that the original glucostatic theory is inadequate. Diabetes mellitus, which is caused by insufficient secretion of the hormone insulin, is characterized by high levels of blood glucose. If the original glucostatic theory were correct, diabetics would have poor appetites. Instead, they show unusually strong appetites. In spite of high blood-glucose levels, diabetics' cells do not extract enough glucose from the bloodstream. Thus, the initiation of eating appears to be more closely related to glucose utilization than to absolute levels of blood glucose.

Glucose utilization is reflected by the difference between the glucose levels of the arteries, which carry blood to the cells, and of the veins, which carry blood away from the cells. High glucose utilization results in large arterio-venous glucose differences which signal the initiation of eating. Low glucose utilization is reflected in low arterio-venous glucose differences which signal the termination of eating. While there is evidence for this theory, there are also some contradictory results. For example, direct injection of glucose into the hypothalamus does not induce termination of eating in food-deprived subjects.

According to the glucostatic view, the initiation of eating is triggered by low glucose utilization and the termination of eating is triggered by high glucose utilization.

7.6 Lipostatic monitoring

The theory of lipostatic monitoring, which was developed by Kennedy, maintains that body weight is monitored via information about the state of body fat deposits. Since fat deposits are not richly supplied by nerves, it seems likely that their state is reflected in a blood-borne message related to fat utilization. Circulating lipids, which are a direct product of fat metabolism, may be involved here. Because fat deposits change only relatively slowly, lipostatic monitoring seems particularly suitable as a long-term regulatory device, perhaps acting together with other shorter-term factors such as temperature and glucose utilization.

The levels of lipids in the blood are an index of fat utilization.

7.7 The brain and body-weight regulation

In the preceding sections we examined a number of possible cues which indicate the state of an organism's energy-balance equation. To translate these signals into the appropriate regulatory behaviours, certain areas of the brain must be activated. Traditionally, emphasis has been placed on the role of various brain "centres" in the regulatory behaviour. In particular, the hypothalamus has frequently been described as a functional mosaic of small, discrete centres for hunger, thirst, satiety, sex and other motivational functions. However, the functional mosaic view is deficient in at least three major respects. First, it overlooks the important role of many other areas of the brain. In an evolutionary sense it would not be very adaptive to develop an organism with all of its "functional eggs" in one small basket, the hypothalamus.

The hypothalamus is neither the anatomical nor functional mosaic that it is frequently described as being.

Second, anatomical studies indicate that, structurally, the hypothalamus is not characterized by clearly defined groups of cells. Various hypothalamic subdivisions merge gradually with each other, and many hypothalamic axons and nerve terminals derive from cell bodies located in other areas of the brain, particularly the mid-brain.

Third, at a functional level, the results of experiments involving direct electrical or chemical stimulation of the hypothalamus do not support the notion of discrete functional compartmentalization. For example, it is clear that stimulation of the hypothalamus may directly elicit eating, drinking and copulation. However, on the basis of electrode location alone, it is not possible to predict which of the numerous behaviours will be elicited. The concept of a functional mosaic has gradually given way to the notion that the hypothalamus is part of a complex and structurally diffuse brain system involved in the modulation of many behaviours.

7.8 The role of the hypothalamus

During the 19th century a number of physicians reported patients suffering from dramatic changes in body weight resulting from tumours near the hypothalamus. The tumours caused voracious eating (hyperphagia) which often led to a doubling of body weight. Since the tumours usually damaged the pituitary gland, which is located immediately below the hypothalamus, it was suggested that the tumours may have stimulated the release of excessive quantities of pituitary growth hormone. However, the patients did not grow into giants. Instead, they grew out into "blobs". The problem was not simply excessive size, it was gross obesity.

Damage to the ventromedial hypothalamic nucleus increases food intake as well as reactivity to many other stimuli.

Damage to the lateral hypothalamic area decreases food intake as well as reactivity to many other stimuli.

The controversy about whether the hyperphagia and obesity were caused by damage to the pituitary or to the adjacent hypothalamus was not resolved until the development of stereotaxic surgical techniques in the 1920s (see 2.3). In experimental animals, selective stereotaxically guided destruction of either the pituitary or hypothalamus showed that pituitary damage by itself did not produce hyperphagia or obesity. It was the hypothalamic damage which produced the hyperphagia and obesity. In particular, a group of cell-bodies, or nucleus, situated near the base (ventral part) at the middle (medial part) of the hypothalamus was implicated in the hyperphagia and obesity. This group of cells is referred to as the ventromedial hypothalamic nucleus.

Because damage to the ventromedial hypothalamic nucleus resulted in excessive eating, it was thought that the brain-damaged animal did not experience satiety. For this reason the ventromedial hypothalamic nucleus is often referred to as a "satiety centre". This was supported by reports that electrical stimulation of the ventromedial hypothalamic nucleus could stop eating (that is, apparently elicit satiety) in a food-deprived rat.

Complementing these findings were results from similar experimental manipulations of an adjacent part of the hypothalamus called the lateral hypothalamic area. Destruction of this area caused a reduction in eating (hypophagia) or, in extreme cases, its elimination (aphagia). The reduction in food intake produced weight losses and in extreme cases the rats starved to death. Conversely, when the lateral hypothalamus was electrically stimulated through implanted electrodes, voracious eating was produced even in fully satiated subjects.

The interpretation of the results followed the same logic as for the ventromedial hypothalamic nucleus. It was assumed that the lack of eating following destruction of the lateral hypothalamic area and the voracious eating following its stimulation indicated that the lateral hypothalamic area was a "hunger centre" which acted in a manner complementary to the ventromedial hypothalamic nucleus "satiety centre". This theory of hypothalamic function is called the dual centres hypothesis.

Before offering alternative interpretations of the above observations, let us consider some aspects of the empirical foundations of the dual centres hypothesis. The most ambiguous aspect of these results is the reduction in eating produced by stimulation of the ventromedial hypothalamic nucleus or destruction of the lateral hypothalamic area.

It is an important general principle of neuroscience research that reducing the vigour of any behaviour does not necessarily reflect a specific inhibition of behaviour but, instead, may be due to general disturbances. For example, stepping on the tail of a cat while it is eating will terminate its eating quickly and dramatically. However, to conclude that the cat's tail has receptors for terminating eating would be wrong.

Lest this example be considered too far-fetched, there are many experiments that show that electrical stimulation of the ventromedial hypothalamic nucleus, which terminates eating, may also cause disturbances in almost any behaviour. Similarly, destruction of the lateral hypothalamic area, besides reducing eating, causes major deficits in many sensory and motor functions. Similar sensorimotor deficits may be produced by selective neurotoxic destruction (see 2.4) of the dopamine neurons which pass through the lateral hypothalamus.

The facilitation of eating produced by lesions of the ventromedial hypothalamic nucleus or stimulation of the lateral hypothalamic area is less likely to be an artifact. However, even these results should be interpreted with caution since recent experiments with rats indicate that a mild tail pinch can elicit eating and drinking. Consequently, some of the eating produced by other experimental manipulations, such as destruction of the ventromedial hypothalamic nucleus or stimulation of the lateral hypothalamic area may reflect a response to mildly stressful events. It has been suggested that eating induced in rats by the tail pinch method may be a useful model of stress-induced obesity in humans.

As described above, the effects of destruction of the lateral hypothalamic area or ventromedial hypothalamic nucleus have usually been interpreted in terms of a reduction in hunger and satiety respectively. Since motivational concepts such as "hunger" and "satiety" cannot be observed directly, it may be more useful to approach this problem in terms of regulation of an objectively measurable variable. Rephrased this way, the traditional view has been that hypothalamic lesions interfere with the organism's ability to regulate its body weight.

Recently, Keesey and colleagues have approached this problem differently. They noted that rats never really recover from hypothalamic lesions. The changes in body weight appear to be permanent. More important, rats that have incurred destruction of either the ventromedial hypothalamic nucleus or the lateral hypothalamic area will actively resist attempts at helping them re-establish their "normal" weight. For example, once an animal with ventromedial hypothalamic lesions has reached its final level of obesity, it is possible to starve it back to its preoperative (i.e. normal) level of body weight. However, as soon as the starvation is discontinued, the rat will rapidly overeat its way back to its former obesity.

Similarly, a rat made obese by destruction of the ventromedial hypothalamic nucleus can be force-fed to make it still more obese. However, as soon as the force-feeding is discontinued the

The active defence of 'abnormal' body weights produced by hypothalamic lesions suggests an alteration in body-weight set-points.

rat will respond by fasting until it re-establishes its former lower level of obesity. Likewise, force-feeding a rat made thin by destruction of the lateral hypothalamic area will cause it to eventually regain its "normal" weight. However, as soon as the force-feeding is stopped, the rat will fast until its former emaciated weight level is re-established.

The active defence of body-weight changes resulting from hypothalamic destruction suggest that the obesity or emaciation following hypothalamic destruction may not be due to an inability to regulate body weight. Instead, these data suggest essentially unimpaired regulation about an altered set-point. In this light aphagia or hyperphagia do not represent a loss of neural control, but rather are purposeful changes in eating directed at maintaining an altered body weight set-point. It should be stressed that the lateral hypothalamic lesions which lower the body weight set-point are rather small. Larger lesions may produce a true loss of neural control of regulation, but since they also seriously disturb many sensory and motor functions it is not certain that the weight loss represents a primary impairment of weight regulation.

7.9 New peripheral theories

Theories of body-weight regulation in the early part of this century stressed the importance of peripheral cues in the initiation of eating and drinking (see 7.2). However, gut rumblings and a dry mouth were soon shown to be neither necessary nor sufficient for either eating or drinking. Moreover, peripheral theories were inconsistent with evidence which showed that a variety of central nervous system manipulations could dramatically alter both eating and drinking.

Recently there has been a renewed interest in the influence of peripheral physiological events on the regulation of body weight. New peripheral theories stress that hunger and consequent eating behaviour reflect the levels of immediately utilizable energy sources. The pivotal organ in energy utilization is the liver. It converts the major energy stores (fat) into appropriate fuels for the rest of the body. Normally, the liver draws on reserves so that metabolic fuels are maintained at a relatively constant level. In addition, the liver directs the break-down of newly ingested food so that appropriate amounts are converted to glycogen, whereas the remainder is stored as fat.

If the delicate metabolic balance is upset so that the liver shifts an abnormally large proportion of newly ingested nutrients to the fat stores, then fat stores will increase in size even if normal food intake is maintained. However, under the above circumstances normal food intake is not maintained, probably for the

The liver is the pivotal peripheral organ in energy utilization.

following reason. The shift of energy disposition towards fat storage results in a corresponding shortage of immediately utilizable fuels (glucose, ketones, and free fatty acids). This shortage generates hunger and, if food is available, the organism will over-eat.

The tendency to convert energy sources preferentially to fat, plus increased eating, results in the rapid development of obesity. According to this view body weight as such is not regulated. Instead, body weight is seen as an incidental by-product of the balancing of the peripheral metabolic equation.

The above approach can also be used to account for the reduction in food intake and body weight produced by lateral hypothalamic lesions. In this case the metabolic error consists of the tendency to convert energy input preferentially to immediately utilizable energy. The result would be a gradual depletion in fat stores, aggravated by reduced eating due to chronically low hunger. This, together with the major sensory and motor deficits produced by lateral hypothalamic lesions, would result in an overall disability which could easily be lethal.

7.10 The neurochemistry of body-weight regulation

The small size and lack of anatomical differentiation of the hypothalamus have contributed to the general failure to localize its many functions anatomically. Consequently, interest has focused on other organizational principles.

Neurons communicate with each other by means of neurotransmitter substances of which there is a substantial number, both proven and suspected. Recent neuroanatomical techniques have made it possible to plot the location in the brain of those neuron systems which use a particular transmitter substance (see 2.1). This technique involves treating brain tissue so that the transmitter chemicals fluoresce when viewed through a special microscope. The procedure is called *fluorescence histochemistry*.

In traditional neuroanatomy, cell groups have been distinguished by other means such as shape, size and density since it was not possible to determine the nature of the transmitter in a particular cell. The histochemical classification system organizes the brain into neuron systems on the basis of their neurotransmitter.

The importance of chemospecific systems is demonstrated by techniques that can specifically enhance or disrupt them. For example, minute quantities of certain neurotransmitters can be injected directly into relatively discrete areas of the brain through a surgically implanted *cannula*. Studies show that the closely related neurotransmitters noradrenalin (norepinephrine), adrenalin (epinephrine), and dopamine significantly increase food intake when administered at a variety of hypothalamic sites. The effects can be blocked by prior injections of agents that normally block transmission in adrenergic neurons.

It appears that the neural systems involved in body-weight regulation are subject to multiple regulatory factors, each characterized by functional, anatomical and neurochemical interaction and redundancy. This "fail safe" system emphasizes the importance of these regulatory mechanisms in the maintenance of life.

This discussion of the neurochemistry of body-weight regulation is necessarily abbreviated. Traditional phrases like "eating is under noradrenergic control" are oversimplifications, as are the earlier notions of eating "centres" in the hypothalamus. As research proceeds, it becomes more apparent that, at the neurochemical level, each behaviour is characterized by a delicate interplay between a number of transmitter systems. This is meant not to intimidate the reader, but to avoid the common pitfall of providing facile answers where questions are more appropriate.

7.11 Body weight, energy balance and dieting

Traditionally, the major emphasis in body-weight regulation has been placed on energy (food) intake. It is widely thought that obesity is caused by over-eating. The corollary of this belief is that obesity is eliminated by under-eating. Thus it may come as a surprise that no one has ever been able to convincingly demonstrate that obese people do actually over-eat. Certainly there are some obese people who over-eat, but there are many who clearly do not over-eat. Conversely, there are some skinny people who under-eat, but there are also many who eat normal or even excessive amounts of food.

It will likely come as less of a surprise that obesity is not eliminated by under-eating. There are abundant data showing that weight reducing diets do not work. The probability of achieving and maintaining a substantial weight loss by dieting is remarkably low. All of these findings suggest that food intake is a rather poor predictor of body weight. Clearly then, there is something fundamentally wrong with traditional views of body-weight regulation.

The major error in traditional views of body-weight regulation is the general failure to consider the role of energy expenditure. According to the laws of thermodynamics, if energy input is not fully reflected in body weight an adjustment in energy expenditure must have taken place. Obesity can be profitably viewed as a problem of energy balance. When energy input is different from energy expenditure, there is an energy

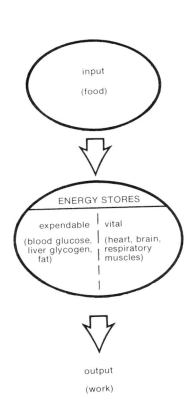

The metabolic equation.

imbalance. Positive energy balance will increase energy storage (body weight), whereas negative energy balance will decrease energy storage.

One reason that the energy expenditure element of the energy balance equation has received little experimental attention is that it is very difficult to measure. In contrast, energy input (food intake) and body weight are relatively easy to measure. Since all of the energy we expend depends on the combination of simple energy sources with oxygen, total energy expenditure is reflected in heat production and oxygen consumption. However, techniques of calorimetry and respirometry are only now becoming sufficiently adequate to accurately measure energy expenditure on a routine basis. Consequently, in the near future we should see dramatic advances in our understanding of energy balance.

Energy expenditure is a very important, yet neglected, component of the energy-balance equation.

Most of our energy (approximately 80%) is automatically expended in the maintenance of body temperature, muscle tone, tissue repair, circulation of the blood, respiration, etc. However, the amount of this unavoidable physiological cost of living which is called *basal metabolism* may vary considerably. The problem is that as yet we know very little about what causes shifts in basal metabolism. This, as we will see below, may well be the major missing key in our understanding of how to alter body weight.

Basal metabolism is the unavoidable physiological cost of living.

When sufficient energy input (food) is not available our bodies attempt to conserve energy by reducing their energy output. Conversely, in response to excess energy input our bodies become energetically wasteful and increase their energy output by increasing radiated heat. This thermal blowoff of excess energy, which is called *luxuskonsumption*, is facilitated by a special type of tissue called *brown fat*. Thus we see that the body automatically compensates for changes in energy input by changing energy output. It is reasonable to assume that such regulatory changes in energy output serve the purpose of defending body weight. If body weight is an actively defended parameter, then changing body weight really involves defeating our own regulatory mechanisms. One would expect this to be difficult if not impossible, and the general failure of weight-altering diets supports this view (see below).

The dissipation of excess energy intake is facilitated by brown fat cells.

This is all bad news for truly obese dieters. These considerations suggest that the body responds to dieting with regulatory mechanisms that have evolved over millions of years. The body "sees" dieting as starvation and responds in the most adaptive way by conserving energy. An important question that has not yet been adequately answered is how much energy input restriction is required to trigger the reduction in energy expenditure. Since the reduction in energy expenditure may not occur immediately, it may be possible for some people to alter their body weight by 5% or even 10% by dieting. It may even be possible to maintain such a weight loss on a long-term basis. The good news is that most dieters would be quite content with a

The body responds to dieting as starvation and not as a means to a more beautiful and healthy self.

5–10% loss in body weight. Further good news is that such weight loss does not require the use of any fad diet. It is simply a matter of reducing energy intake. The best way to do this is by eating boring, unpalatable food. That is, in effect, what most fad diets amount to. In the face of unvarying and unpalatable food, energy intake declines.

The role of exercise in energy balance is poorly understood.

It also seems that exercise may not be a good way to lose weight. Exercise is unquestionably good for one's general health and well-being, but it may add remarkably little to overall energy expenditure. For example, three one-hour sessions of competition squash would add only a fraction of 1% to the player's weekly energy expenditure. Very few people have the opportunity or inclination to produce significant long-term increases in their energy expenditure by exercise. However, there is a possibility that the increased energy expenditure produced by exercise may persist well beyond the exercise session itself. If this can be shown then exercise may indeed have a significant role to play in regulating body weight.

The health liability associated with obesity is generally far overstated.

For the truly obese person the picture is rather bleak. The bright side of the picture is that obesity is not likely to be nearly the health liability that it is usually claimed to be. Few would argue that obesity is good for you, yet the health liability associated with obesity is certainly not sufficient to engender the state of near panic that it often does.

On the other hand, dieting is certainly stressful, and stress is unquestionably a health hazard (see 9.5). In some cases dieting may well turn out to be another case where the cure is more dangerous than the disease. The dark side of the picture is that the probability of achieving a weight loss much greater than 10% is very low. In one recent study of grossly obese people who underwent hospitalization involving long periods of semi- and total starvation, less than half could reduce to within 30% of their "ideal" body weight (still a grossly obese weight). Two years later only 6 of the 206 dieters were still within the 30% of ideal weight range. The great diet success stories which appear continually in advertisements are simply not representative of a typical person. Such misleading half-truths are usually fostered by people who are selling diets or diet products. At the moment the diet consumer appears to be buying little more than false hopes and disillusionment.

Diets are not nearly as successful as those who sell them would have us believe.

People go to bizarre and dangerous extremes to defeat their own physiological regulatory mechanisms.

The desperation felt by the obese is well reflected in the bizarre lengths to which they will go in order to lose weight. For example, many people have had their jaws wired shut so that it is impossible for them to eat other than from a straw. The logic behind this is that excessive eating is a learned response to stress and that the jaw wiring forces the patient to learn a new coping mechanism. Whereas the jaw wiring is safe and it does produce significant weight loss, on removing the wiring the patients almost invariably regain their lost weight. Consequently, just like so many other weight-reducing procedures, the usefulness of jaw wiring is negated by its failure to produce long-term weight loss.

Another more drastic, surgical approach to weight reduction is the intestinal bypass. This operation "short-circuits" most of the small intestine. By reducing the effective area of the intestines to which food is exposed, the advocates of this procedure claim a reduction in energy absorption. It offers the attractive possibility of having your cake without its appearing on your waistline. In one recent study of 10 patients, two demanded that the bypass be reversed, one committed suicide and two more died as a result of the operation. Irrespective of the results of the other five patients, such data constitute a strong indictment of intestinal bypass surgery.

7.12 Osmotic monitoring of fluid balance

Energy balance and fluid balance are to some extent inter-dependent. This is indicated by the fact that severely food-deprived animals usually voluntarily restrict their water intake. However, in spite of this interdependency there is a great deal of evidence suggesting that fluid balance is regulated by a different set of cues involving different neural mechanisms.

Cells are both filled with fluid, intracellular fluid, and bathed in a fluid medium, extracellular fluid. Severe water deprivation reduces the volume of the extracellular fluid. This results in increased extracellular sodium ion (Na^+) concentration. Since the cell membrane is relatively impermeable to Na^+, there is a tendency for intracellular fluid to move out of the cell to restore the original concentration difference. This fluid movement, or osmosis, results in cell shrinkage which is detected by special-ized hypothalamic receptor cells called *osmoreceptors*. Osmotic monitoring explains the occurrence of increased drinking after a salty meal, even though salt intake does not produce a fluid deficit. Because the drinking is produced by increased osmotic pressure, it is called hyperosmotic drinking. The major defect of the osmotic monitoring theory is that cellular shrinkage occurs only with abnormal salt intake or extreme water deprivation, whereas most drinking takes place under far less extreme conditions.

Salty foods produce thirst because they cause cell shrinkage.

7.13 Volume monitoring of fluid balance

Although moderate water deprivation produces drinking, it does not cause significant cell shrinkage. Moderate water deprivation does, however, result in a small decrease in the total volume of extracellular fluids, particularly that of the blood. This state of

Thirst is most commonly produced by a minute decrease in extracellular fluid volume.

decreased extracellular fluid volume is called *hypovolemia*. A decrease in blood volume results in a decrease in blood pressure which is detected by sensitive peripheral pressure receptors which relay their message to the brain.

Because the kidneys regulate much of our water excretion, it is not surprising that they are also involved in the mediation of hypovolemic drinking. Decreased blood pressure causes the kidney to release an enzyme called renin which converts a normal blood-borne protein into angiotensin II. Angiotensin II acts directly on the brain to elicit drinking (see 7.14). Supporting this theory is the observation that blood loss, for example in an accident or haemorrhage, is a strong drink-inducing stimulus.

7.14 The neurochemistry of fluid balance

Drinking can be produced by intracerebral injections of acetylcholine or angiotensin II.

Grossman first showed that acetylcholine could elicit vigorous drinking when applied through cannulas to the hypothalamus. Other researchers have verified Grossman's results, and have further shown that cholinergic drinking can be produced at many sites within the limbic system. Perhaps the most potent drink-inducing chemical is angiotensin II. In contrast to the anatomical diversity of cholinergic drinking, angiotensin II drinking is generally only elicited from cannulas located in the anterior hyothalamus or from two highly specialized organs near the cerebral ventricles. The subfornical organ and the organum vasculosum of the lamina terminals are equisitely sensitive to blood-borne angiotensin II. As little as 5×10^{-15} g of angiotensin II applied to the organum vasculosum of the lamina terminalis produces vigorous and long-lasting drinking. Conversely, destruction of these two organs produces severe, even fatal, dehydration.

7.15 Temperature regulation

The human body temperature set-point (37°C) is far closer to the lethal upper limit (44°C) than to the lethal lower limit (16°C).

Virtually every chemical reaction necessary for the maintenance of life is temperature dependent. As temperature decreases, the rates of the reactions become progressively slower, until eventually they stop altogether and the organism dies. As temperature increases, the rates of many reactions increase, but at the same time the proteins, which are the basic building blocks of life, begin to break down. At high temperatures death results from the fact that the rate of protein destruction far exceeds the organism's restorative abilities. There are reports of humans recovering from internal body temperatures as low as 16°C and as high as 44°C. Note that since the set-point body temperature for humans is 37°C, the above extremes represent a downward excursion of 21°C and an upward excursion of only 7°C. Why our temperature set-point is so near the lethal upper limit remains unanswered.

The relatively narrow range of permissible body temperatures contrasts sharply with the extreme range of environmental temperatures in which mammals can operate. This attests to the efficiency of our thermoregulatory mechanisms. Astronauts have endured external temperatures of 300°C when heavily clothed, and 250°C when naked, temperatures well above those required to fry bacon.

Our ability to maintain a constant body temperature (homeothermia, from the Greek, meaning "same temperature") in the face of radical changes in environmental temperatures, gives us greater independence of the environment than is possible for non-homeothermic organisms. Organisms whose body temperature closely reflects that of the environment are called poikilothermic or "cold-blooded".

Homeotherms have a much higher degree of environmental independence. than poikilotherms.

Much of the behaviour of poikilotherms is directed towards maintaining themselves in an environment of suitable temperature. At high temperatures poikilotherms must seek shelter, whereas at low temperatures they become inactive or hibernate. The difference in environmental dependence of homeothermic and poikilothermic organisms shows the behavioural results of physiological characteristics. Homeothermia results in greater mobility and more varied behaviour.

7.16 Production, conservation and loss of heat

Before considering the control of thermoregulation by the central nervous system we need to discuss briefly the physiological mechanisms by which we produce, conserve or lose body heat. While this discussion will focus on the physiological mechanisms of thermoregulation, it must be remembered that thermoregulation is not only physiological, but also behavioural. Under normal circumstances, for example, if we are too cold we can put on more clothes, seek shelter, or light a fire. Conversely, if we are too warm we can shed clothes, fan ourselves, or take a swim.

	Thermoregulatory Mechanisms
HEAT PRODUCTION	shivering, increased muscle tone, increased metabolism
HEAT CONSERVATION	constriction of surface blood vessels, decreased respiratory volume
HEAT LOSS	sweating, decreased muscle tone, dilation of surface blood vessels, increased respiratory volume, decreased metabolism

7.17 The brain and thermoregulation

In thermoregulation, more so than with any other regulatory system, the principal focus of attention has been, and still is, the hypothalamus. However, there is evidence which increasingly implicates other areas of the brain in thermoregulation. The brain must receive some message concerning the current state of the system. This is the sensory component of the system. Then, the sensory input must be compared with the set-point to determine whether a thermoregulatory response is necessary. This is the integration component. If required, the integrator must initiate the appropriate regulatory response. This is the effector component. Since we know that some parts of the brain are relatively specialized to serve sensory, integrative and effector functions, it is clear that a regulatory system will inevitably involve several different parts of the brain.

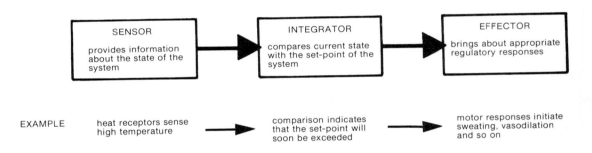

Flow diagram of a generalized regulatory system and an example of thermoregulation.

7.18 Hypothalamic mechanisms

Destruction of the anterior hypothalamus destroys the ability to cope with heat stress, but it does not affect the ability to cope with cold stress. Conversely, destruction of the posterior hypothalamus destroys the ability to cope with cold stress without affecting the response to heat stress.

Complementary data come from studies in which hypothalamic function has been altered by electrical stimulation through implanted electrodes. Electrical stimulation of anterior hypothalamus results in decreased body temperature and a suppression of shivering in the cold. Electrical stimulation of the posterior hypothalamus results in increased body temperature and shivering, even in a warm environment. These results indicate that the anterior hypothalamus facilitates heat loss, and the posterior hypothalamus facilitates heat production.

7.19 Ionic balance as the basis of the set-point

Of great interest in thermoregulatory research is Myers' identification of a potential physiological basis for the set-point for body temperature. Myers presents evidence that the temperature set-point is maintained by a balance between sodium (Na^+) and calcium (Ca^{2+}) ions in a restricted area of the posterior hypothalamus. Application of Na^+ ions increases body temperature, whereas application of Ca^{2+} ions to the same site decreases body temperature. The changes did not occur in response to other ions, such as potassium (K^+) or magnesium (Mg^{2+}), nor if the Na^+ or Ca^{2+} ions were applied to other parts of the hypothalamus.

Similar temperature changes can be brought about by electrical stimulation or by intrahypothalamic injections of many other substances. Nevertheless, Myers claims that the set-point is determined by the ion balance and not by other means. He notes that the subject will actively defend the ion-induced changes over a long period, whereas other hypothalamic manipulations simply impair regulation.

Monkeys will actively defend an ionically altered set-point.

Note the similarity between Myers' logic and that of Keesey in his studies of the set-point for body weight. For example, Keesey's fat rats would repeatedly defend their obesity by appropriately increasing or decreasing their food intake in response to starvation or force-feeding.

Myers demonstrated a similar defence of an altered temperature set-point by increasing the body temperature of a monkey to the dangerously high level of 41°C by removing Ca^{2+} ions from the hypothalamus. The high temperature could be maintained for hours, with the monkey showing none of the responses such as panting, vasodilation, and sweating that would normally occur.

However, if its body temperature were further increased by other means, the regulatory responses would promptly appear, lowering body temperature, but only to 41°C. Conversely, even though the animal was clearly in a state of thermal stress, lowering its temperature by a drink of cold water resulted in the prompt appearance of shivering and vasoconstriction which raised its temperature again to 41°C.

Questions

1 Consider the possibility that the changes in eating following various brain manipulations are artifactual.
2 Is body weight really regulated at all?
3 Do the changes in eating following hypothalamic lesions indicate a loss of neural control?
4 Discuss the social and physiological pros and cons of dieting.

5 Why should body temperature be so closely regulated?
6 Why is our body temperature set-point so close to the lethal upper limit?
7 Describe how Myers has isolated the mechanism of the set-point.

Further Readings

Dawson, T.J. Kangaroos. *Scientific American*, 1977, **237** (2), 78–89.

Garrow, J.S. *Energy Balance and Obesity in Man*. Amsterdam, Elsevier. 1978.

Fitzsimons, J.T. Angiotensin stimulation of the central nervous system. *Reviews of Physiology, Biochemistry and Pharmacology*, 1980, **87**, 117–167.

Jones, W.P.T. *Research on Obesity. A Report of the DHSS/MRC group*. London, Her Majesty's Stationery Office. 1976.

Powers, P.S. *Obesity: The Regulation of Body Weight*. Baltimore, Md., Williams & Wilkins. 1980.

Rolls, B.J., Rowe, E.A. and Turren, R.C. Persistant obesity in rats following a period of mixed, high energy diet. *Journal of Physiology*, 1980, **298**, 415–427.

Rothwell, N.J. and Stock, M.J. Regulation of energy balance in two models of reversible obesity in the rat. *Journal of Comparative and Physiological Psychology*, 1979, **93**, 1024–1034.

Wurtman, R.J. and Wurtman, J.J. (Eds) *Nutrition and the Brain*, Vol. 3. New York, Raven Press. 1979.

8
Reinforcement Mechanisms

8.1 Introduction

The concept of reinforcement or reward is basic to an explanation of why the full range of behaviours possible to an animal do not occur with equal probability under all circumstances. From a wide range of possibilities, reinforcement is important in determining which responses will be learned and will increase in probability. For example, if a rat is placed in a maze with cheese in the goal box, changes occur in the rat's behaviour over repeated trials. Initially the rat wanders about aimlessly. This random behaviour continues until the rat finds the cheese. Subsequently when the rat is placed in the maze, its behaviour becomes progressively less random. Responses that do not facilitate finding the cheese are gradually eliminated. Eventually the rat negotiates the maze in an errorless and efficient way.

Reinforcement explains why some things are learned and some are not.

The change in behaviour is an example of learning which took place because the maze-running behaviour was reinforced by the tasty piece of cheese. We could say also, although it involves more inference, that eating the cheese was pleasurable. Theorists have debated the relative contribution to behaviour of learning as opposed to genetic influences, but few would dispute the importance of learning in the understanding of behaviour. Further, it is clear that a large amount of learning involves specifiable sources of reinforcement.

A conclusive experiment to demonstrate the relative effects of heredity and environment would involve two groups, one which had heredity but no environment, and the other with environment but no heredity.

The rat in the maze illustrates learning reinforced by something pleasurable. Learning can also be reinforced by avoidance of, or escape from, something unpleasant such as electric shock. Thus the concept of reinforcement is associated with pleasure, displeasure, and other emotional or affective states. We shall

examine the physiology of the neural systems mediating reinforcement and emotion in Chapter 9. In Chapter 11 we shall see
how this area of research has provided information about the
mode of action of psychotherapeutic drugs.

8.2 The neural basis of reward

In 1954, almost by accident, Olds and Milner made observations
which led to a new area of research in the neurosciences. They
were examining the effects on rats of electrical stimulation of the
brain through surgically implanted electrodes. At first the brain
stimulation produced no change in the rat's behaviour. However,
with repeated testing the rat began to spend most of its time on
the part of the table top where it received the brain stimulation.
Note the similarity between this observation and the example of
maze learning described above. With repeated testing the rat's
behaviour in both cases became progressively less random. The
difference is that in the maze the change was brought about by
a specifiable reward, cheese, whereas on the table top the change
was the result of the electrical stimulation of a small area of the
brain. The intensity of these stimulating impulses is often so low
that they cannot be detected by the external senses. In other
words, brain stimulation can produce a reinforcing effect even
though it completely by-passes all known sensory mechanisms.
These observations raised the exciting prospect that Olds and
Milner had intervened directly in the brain mechanisms involved in the experience of reward.

The reinforcing effect of electrical stimulation of the brain is
demonstrated by the fact that an organism will learn any arbitrary response when it is consistently followed by brain stimulation. This phenomenon is referred to as self-stimulation. The
generality of the self-stimulation phenomenon is indicated by its
demonstration in every species studied to date, from goldfish to
humans.

The strength of brain stimulation as a reinforcer is so great
that animals may self-stimulate to the point of physical exhaustion. In a frequently cited study, rats were reported to self-
stimulate so vigorously and compulsively that they ignored basic
biological needs and virtually starved themselves to death. This
example has been used to conjure up a grim spectre of legions of
electronic "zombies" controlled by brain stimulation. In fact, the
self-starvation phenomenon is quite atypical and occurs only
under a restricted set of conditions.

8.3 Anatomical locus of reinforcement effects

Electrical stimulation of some brain areas yields positive reinforcement effects, whereas stimulation of other areas appears to

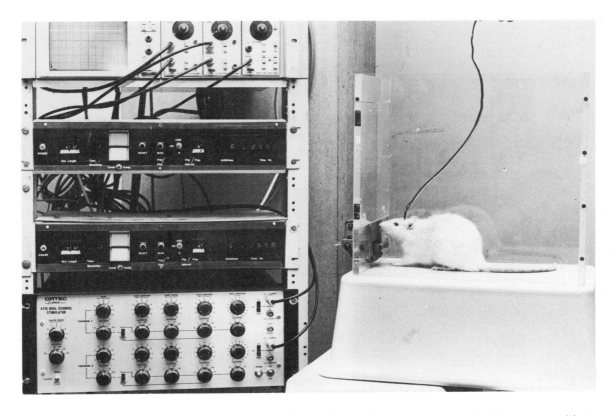

A rat self-stimulating in a lever-press chamber. Pressing the lever produces a short (usually 0.5 sec) train of brain stimulation. The equipment at the left is for recording behaviour and monitoring the brain stimulation.

have no reinforcing effects. Although the term "pleasure centre" is still used, more than 25 years of research have shown that reinforcing effects are not centred at all, but rather are found in anatomically diffuse groups of structures. Once again we see that brain function is rarely organized in terms of localized centres and that the concept of anatomically extensive systems is more consistent with the available evidence.

Traditionally, stimulation of a loose fibre system that courses through the lateral hypothalamus has been considered to produce the strongest reinforcement effects. This system of fibres is called the medial forebrain bundle. The cell bodies of most neurons of the medial forebrain bundle are located either in the brain stem or in the forebrain. As would be expected, stimulation of the sites of origin of the median forebrain bundle neurons is also reinforcing. Whereas the forebrain reinforcement effects are usually less potent than those obtained from lateral hypothalamic electrodes, some of the brain stem sites, particularly those in the ventral tegmentum and the substantia nigra, are at least as potent as those in the lateral hypothalamus.

Although the medial forebrain bundle is a particularly good site for obtaining self-stimulation, there are many other effective brain areas as well.

Reinforcement effects may also be produced well outside the medial forebrain bundle. In particular, consider the case of the hypothalamic paraventricular system which, as its name suggests, runs along the most medial aspect of the hypothalamus immediately next to the third ventricle. The paraventricular system has been said to be an aversion system which acts in a reciprocal or push–pull manner with the medial forebrain bundle reward system. These two systems are frequently described as respectively constituting a "stop" and "go" system for behaviour. The evidence most commonly cited to support this view is that animals with medial forebrain bundle electrodes will work to initiate brain stimulation, whereas animals with paraventricular system electrodes will work to escape brain stimulation.

Although the above view is simple and appealing it is almost certainly incorrect. This is indicated by the demonstration that, if given the opportunity, animals with paraventricular electrodes will initiate the same brain stimulation that they will escape. Conversely, if given the opportunity, animals with medial forebrain bundle electrodes will escape the same brain stimulation that they will initiate.

8.4 Measuring the motivational properties of brain stimulation

The fact that animals initiate brain stimulation and then, after receiving a certain amount of brain stimulation, they escape it is easily demonstrated in a shuttle box. In the shuttle box the animal may initiate brain stimulation simply by interrupting a photobeam at one end of the box. Once initiated, the animal may escape the brain stimulation simply by interrupting a photobeam at the other end of the box.

Many experimenters have found that at virtually any electrode location where the animal will initiate brain stimulation, after receiving about 5–20 seconds of stimulation, it will escape the stimulation. This pattern of initiation followed by escape is referred to as shuttling. The vigour of initiation behaviour, commonly expressed as a latency or rate measure, is usually taken to be an index of the reward value of the brain stimulation. A low latency or high rate to initiate suggests that the brain stimulation is very rewarding. Conversely, a high latency or low rate to initiate brain stimulation suggests a low reward value.

There is far less agreement on how escape from rewarding brain stimulation should be interpreted. Perhaps the most obvious interpretation of the escape behaviour, is that, like any other type of escape behaviour, it indicates aversion. However, there are at least two plausible alternative explanations to account for

The escape from rewarding brain stimulation is subject to several quite different interpretations.

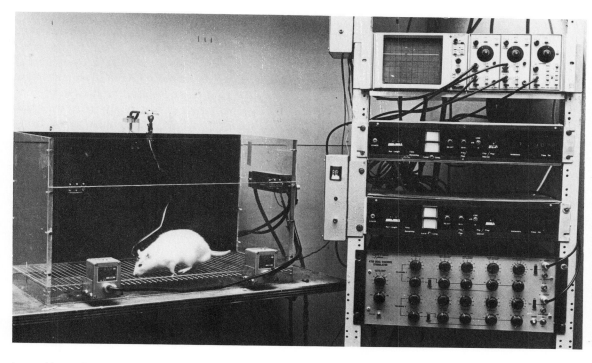

A rat self-stimulating in a shuttle box. Moving to the left side of the box turns on the brain stimulation, whereas moving to the right turns it off. The equipment at the right is for recording behaviour and monitoring the brain stimulation.

the escape from rewarding brain stimulation, neither of which is based upon aversion.

One common interpretation of the escape from rewarding brain stimulation is that the escape takes place simply because long trains of brain stimulation cease to be rewarding. Note that the absence of reward is very different from the presence of an active aversion process.

Another interpretation is based on the common observation that rewarding brain stimulation often directly elicits locomotor behaviour and exploration. According to this view the elicited locomotor behaviour results in escape as an incidental effect of the animal's being very active. Reasonably, the animal then re-initiates the stimulation to reactivate the reward system. This, of course, starts the elicitation process once again and produces shuttling behaviour. The crux of the elicitation hypothesis is that the escape behaviour is reflexively elicited by the brain stimulation and it is not a purposive attempt to terminate the stimulation.

Recent experiments have demonstrated that, whereas the escape from long trains of rewarding brain stimulation is partly elicited and does indicate reward adaptation, there is also a significant aversive component to the stimulation. The inadequacy of the pure elicitation hypothesis was demonstrated by the effects of terminating the brain stimulation automatically, independently of the animal's behaviour. Even in extensively trained rats, eliminating the escape contingency produced an immediate reduction in the escape behaviour. Reinstating the escape contingency produced a rapid return of maximally vigorous escape behaviour. Clearly, the escape from brain stimulation was being reinforced by the termination of brain stimulation. It was not simply elicited by it.

Whereas the above data do show that the escape from rewarding stimulation is not elicited, they still do not constitute adequate proof that the stimulation becomes aversive. If long trains of rewarding brain stimulation really do become aversive, then the animals should not work to initiate such long trains. Or at least they should not work as hard to initiate long trains as they would for shorter trains. If long trains of rewarding brain stimulation simply cease to be as rewarding, then a train of brain stimulation of any length should be at least as rewarding as any shorter lengths. The aversion hypothesis predicts that trains of stimulation beyond a certain length should produce decreased rates to initiate those trains. In contrast, the adaptation hypothesis predicts that increasing train lengths will eventually result in no further increases in initiation rate. If any increase in stimulation train length decreases the rate to initiate stimulation, the decrease must represent the effects of an active aversive process.

Experiments like that described above have shown that, in nearly all rats with lateral hypothalamic electrodes, long stimulation trains are significantly less rewarding than much shorter trains. These findings unequivocally support the aversion hypothesis. However, the length of train required to produce the decrement in initiation rate is usually greater than the animals self-select. In other words, if the animal can escape the brain stimulation and then immediately re-initiate it, it will choose low to medium length trains. Under such conditions it is likely that the escape from rewarding brain stimulation represents an attempt to foil adaptation by never letting it occur. Real aversion is only reflected in the decrease in initiation rates which is produced by much longer trains. Thus, in a sense, all of the above three hypotheses to account for the escape from rewarding brain stimulation are correct. The escape is partly elicited and partly motivated by adaptation of reward and the presence of an active aversive process. The uncontrolled operation of a combination of these three factors has undoubtedly contributed greatly to the confusion that exists in the literature on self-stimulation.

The above considerations suggest that elicitation, adaptation of reward and an active aversive process may all confound the measurement of the rewarding aspect of brain stimulation. There

Depending on the experimental circumstances, the escape from rewarding brain stimulation may indicate aversion, adaptation of reward, or behaviour elicitation.

is another equally important factor that may operate in conjunction with the above confounds. This is the effect of *priming*. Priming is demonstrated by the fact that one train of brain stimulation appears to greatly enhance the performance for subsequent trains of brain stimulation. The analogy is based on the facilitating effects of priming a water pump with a little water. During continuous reinforcement each train of brain stimulation acts *both* to reward the previous response and to prime the next response. The problem this raises is that, if an experimental treatment (say a drug) reduced the rate of self-stimulation, the reduction could represent either a decrease in the rewarding value of the stimulation and/or a decrease in the facilitation produced by priming. The reduced rate could also reflect a simple motor impairment and have nothing to do with either priming or reward.

At the same time, the reduced response rate reduces the total amount of brain stimulation and alters its temporal spacing. This, of course, alters behaviour elicitation, reward adaptation and aversion. The point of this example is to show that in conventional self-stimulation situations any change in the rate of responding could be due to changes in:

The measurement of brain stimulation reward is usually confounded by the numerous other performance-altering properties of the brain stimulation.

- reward strength
- priming
- activity
- behaviour elicitation
- adaptation of reward
- aversion

With so many uncontrolled and poorly understood factors operating it is clearly unjustifiable to assert that a decrease in the rate of self-stimulation indicates a decrease in reward strength. Yet this is just what the great majority of researchers in this area continue to do.

The encouraging aspect of the methodological inadequacies described above is that improvements to self-stimulation measuring techniques may be able to provide information on reward as well as all of the other interesting and generally unexplored aspects of rewarding brain stimulation.

One improved self-stimulation paradigm is an adaptation of the shuttle box procedure described in 8.3 and 8.4. The main inadequacy of the shuttle box as used to date is that both the initiation of and escape from stimulation are subject to continuous reinforcement contingencies. This procedure leads to serious confounds since changes in performance change the total amount and temporal distribution of the brain stimulation.

If the total amount and temporal distribution of the brain stimulation were held constant across a wide range of response rates, then changes in the rate of stimulation initiation and escape would respectively provide relatively unconfounded measures of the initiation and escape performance. A reasonable approximation of this ideal can be achieved in the shuttle box by making both the initation of, and escape from, brain stimulation subject to fixed-interval contingencies. In this situation the first response after a fixed-interval (say 30 secs) initiates the brain stimulation. Then after another fixed interval (say 10 secs) the first response terminates the brain stimulation. Given a minimal level of responding, these contingencies ensure that each animal receives almost identical amounts of brain stimulation under all conditions. Although this paradigm is just beginning to be explored it holds great promise for unravelling some of the complexities of the self-stimulation phenomenon.

8.5 Chemical stimulation of the brain

Neurons communicate with each other by the release of chemical transmitter substances at their synapses. Since electrical stimulation of the brain ultimately produces its rewarding effects by altering chemical transmission, it should be possible to produce reward by administering small amounts of the neurotransmitters to the brain. This can be done directly through surgically implanted cannulas, or indirectly by administering various pharmacological agents into the bloodstream.

Generally, however, peripherally administered neurotransmitters do not reach the brain. Their entry to the brain is prevented by the blood–brain barrier, which protects the brain by restricting the types of molecules that can enter it. The barrier generally blocks large molecules, and most chemical transmitter substances are rather large molecules. However, many substances when administered peripherally do enter the brain where they may then affect neuronal activity by altering chemical transmission. Most of the drugs which affect behaviour, mood, sensation, thought processes and arousal exert their effects by altering synaptic transmission. They are the psychoactive drugs, and this area of research is psychopharmacology.

It should be possible to train animals to self-administer chemicals to the brain in much the same way as they self-administer electrical stimulation. However, the repetitive intracranial administration of chemicals poses some formidable technical problems. For example, the smallest volume of a solution that can be reliably delivered through a cannula is approximately 0.5 microlitres (five millionths of a litre or 0.5 μl). Since the entire volume of one side of the rat hypothalamus is only about 4.0 μl, 8 self-stimulation responses would leave the hypothalamus dripping with fluid. Results obtained under such non-physiological conditions would be difficult to interpret.

The volume limitations can be circumvented by training the animal on a maze learning task which requires only one trial a

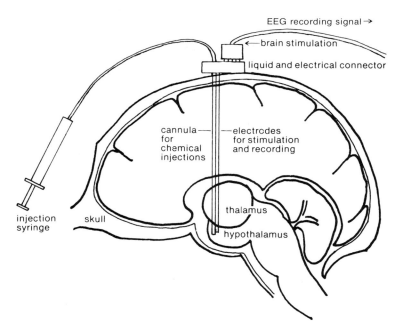

Procedure for chemical and electrical stimulation of the brain with concurrent EEG recording. The combination of a cannula and electrode is referred to as a chemitrode.

day. Recently it has been shown that some rats will consistently choose the arm of a T-maze where noradrenaline is injected into the hypothalamus, whereas other rats will just as reliably avoid that arm. These results suggest that for some rats the noradrenalin injections were rewarding, but for others aversive. The findings indicate that simple statements such as "reinforcement is due to the release of noradrenalin in the hypothalamus" may be serious oversimplifications.

Another self-stimulation procedure involves subjects performing a response reinforced by intravenous drug injection. The applicability of this technique to the problems of human drug abuse is obvious, since many of the more common drugs of abuse such as heroin, morphine and amphetamine are often administered intravenously. Laboratory animals whose blood streams have been surgically connected to a syringe which they can operate by pressing a lever show certain regularities in their drug self-administration behaviour. If the syringe contains an inert fluid, little lever-pressing occurs. However, if a substance such as amphetamine ("speed") is added, the behaviour of the subject rapidly changes. The animal will press the lever repeatedly until some terminal blood level of the drug is reached. Subsequently, lever pressing becomes slower and steadier so that a constant blood level of amphetamine is maintained. If the

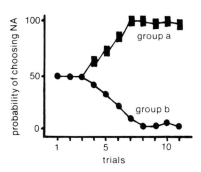

Results of a T-maze experiment with rats. Choosing one arm of the maze resulted in an intracranial injection of noradrenalin. Choosing the other arm resulted in an intracranial injection of inert saline. Group A consistently chose the noradrenalin, whereas group B just as consistently avoided it.

concentration of the injection solution is increased or decreased, the rate of lever-pressing will decrease or increase respectively so that a fairly constant blood level of amphetamine is maintained.

That the reinforcing value of amphetamine may be due to the release of the neurotransmitter dopamine is suggested by two observations. First, the drug pimozide, which is a highly selective dopamine receptor blocker, causes an increase in the rate of amphetamine self-administration, indicating that not enough drug is "getting through" to the critical dopamine receptors. Second, laboratory animals will also self-administer apomorphine which is a relatively specific dopamine receptor stimulant.

8.6 The neurochemistry of reinforcement

It has generally been maintained that hypothalamic stimulation activates the neural systems involved in reward and a variety of affective states. Consequently, self-stimulation experiments have been used widely to evaluate the mode of action of various psychoactive drugs. However, the current literature abounds with contradictions and unsupported speculation. Perhaps because self-stimulation is so easily demonstrated and permits such a high degree of behavioural control, the phenomenon seems to have attracted more than its share of what might be called "neuromythology".

The self-stimulation phenomenon has at various times been related to depression, schizophrenia, anxiety, obesity, anorexia, obsession, sexual deviation, drug addiction, learning and memory. Many of these rather speculative associations derive from observations of the effects of various psychoactive drugs on self-stimulation. For example, it is frequently noted that a drug such as reserpine, which may induce psychiatric depression in humans, depresses self-stimulation. In contrast, it has been claimed that a clinical anti-depressant such as imipramine facilitates self-stimulation.

As the drugs respectively decrease or increase noradrenalin availability, the results have been used to support a noradrenergic theory of reinforcement, and by inference a noradrenergic theory of depression. However, most studies suggest that imipramine and related drugs depress self-stimulation. A drug like amphetamine, which provokes or increases schizophrenic symptoms, increases the vigour of self-stimulation. In contrast, a drug like haloperidol, which decreases schizophrenic symptoms, decreases the vigour of self-stimulation. Since amphetamine and haloperidol respectively increase and decrease dopamine availability, their effects on self-stimulation are said to support a dopaminergic theory of both reward and schizophrenia. Yet, as is the case with anti-depressant drugs, there are also conflicting findings in the case of some dopaminergic manipulations. For example, massive dopamine depletion may have almost no effect on self-stimulation, whereas a dopamine stimulant such as apomorphine may depress self-stimulation.

Interpretation and integration of such conflicting results is complicated by three problems, two methodological and one conceptual. The two methodological difficulties are problems of specificity. One comes from the lack of pharmacological specificity of the drugs, and the other from the lack of behavioural specificity of their effects. The conceptual problem arises from a misunderstanding of how various agents might be expected to affect self-stimulation.

Most drugs affect more than one neurotransmitter system and they may alter transmitter availability in a number of different ways. For example, the anti-depressant imipramine is often used experimentally because of its ability to block the re-uptake of noradrenalin. However, imipramine has a number of other effects. Consequently, even if imipramine reliably facilitated self-stimulation, which is doubtful, to attribute its behavioural effects to the re-uptake blockade of noradrenalin or any other single neurochemical effect is not justified. A similar analysis could be made of most other drugs used in self-stimulation experiments. Since some new and specific drugs are appearing on the market, a few questions of pharmacological specificity may be clarified in the near future.

If a neurochemically selective drug is employed, there remains the problem of behavioural specificity. Does a change in the vigour of self-stimulation represent a change in reward, or does it reflect a non-specific change in activity or reactivity? For example, amphetamine increases the rate of self-stimulation, and is consequently said to increase reward. However, amphetamine appears to increase the vigour of almost all behaviours.

Consider a hungry rat lever-pressing for food. Amphetamine causes a marked increase in the rate of lever-pressing which could be interpreted as reflecting the increased reward value of food. However, amphetamine is a notorious appetite suppressant and while the drugged rats do lever-press more rapidly, indicating increased reward value of food, they ignore the food, indicating reduced reward value of food. Thus increased response vigour does not necessarily indicate reward enhancement.

Conversely, the anti-schizophrenic drug haloperidol reduces the vigour of self-stimulation, but since it is a strong sedative and tends to cause general immobility, it also reduces the vigour of most other responses. Again, it may not be correct to infer a reduction in reward solely on the basis of decreased response vigour. In order to understand clearly drug effects on behaviour, it is necessary to examine the effects of the drug on more than one aspect of the subject's behaviour.

One of the difficulties in determining the neurochemical basis of reward is that nearly all drugs influence more than one neurochemical system.

Some neurochemical effects of imipramine:
- *noradrenalin re-uptake blockade*
- *serotonin re-uptake blockade*
- *dopamine re-uptake blockade*
- *monoamine oxidase inhibition*
- *acetylcholine antagonism*
- *histamine antagonism*

Changes in the vigour of self-stimulation produced by drugs do not necessarily indicate changes in the reward value of the stimulation. The effects could represent general sedative or stimulant effects, as well as the interactions of these effects with the numerous uncontrolled performance-altering effects found in typical test situations.

The question of the general as opposed to the specific reward modulating effects of drugs may be solved by employing a shuttle-box to assess self-stimulation performance. By concurrently measuring both the initiation of, and escape from, brain stimulation, the shuttle-box allows the differentiation of general shifts in the vigour of performance from specific reward modulation effects. For example, in the shuttle-box the anti-schizophrenic agent clozapine decreases the vigour of the initiation behaviour, while leaving the escape behaviour unaffected. Thus we can conclude that clozapine produced a selective reduction of reward without generally disturbing the animal. Conversely, in the shuttle-box amphetamine has been shown to produce a selective increase in the vigour of the initiation behaviour. This allows us to state with more certainty that amphetamine was increasing reward quite apart from its tendency to generally increase the vigour of behaviour. However, even these findings are subject to the confounds which plague all continuous reinforcement self-stimulation findings (see 8.4).

It is worth noting that the specificity of clozapine's effects on self-stimulation is closely paralleled by its clinical specificity. Clozapine reduces schizophrenic symptoms without producing the general disturbances in motor functioning that accompany the administration of traditional anti-schizophrenic drugs such as haloperidol.

The third problem in the interpretation of self-stimulation results derives from some confusion about the way in which various neurochemical changes should be expected to affect performance. It is generally thought that drugs which facilitate monoaminergic transmission facilitate self-stimulation. Apart from the issue of which monoamines are critical, this statement contains an important conceptual error. There are at least four ways of enhancing monoaminergic transmission, and it is not at all clear that they have equivalent effects on self-stimulation.

The data concerning drugs which increase transmitter release are relatively consistent. Release-facilitating agents like amphetamine and cocaine generally enhance reward. The results based on the other three methods of facilitating monoamine effects are more contradictory, with various researchers reporting increased, decreased and unchanged self-stimulation. When a control for behavioural specificity is employed, it appears that the other three methods of increasing monoaminergic availability decrease the vigour of self-stimulation. The paradox is, why should increasing monoaminergic availability one way increase reward, whereas increasing monoaminergic availability other ways appears to reduce reward?

The resolution to the above paradox necessitates consideration of the way in which brain stimulation and the monoaminergic transmission facilitators affect synaptic transmission. When the

Different ways of facilitating mono-aminergic transmission and examples of drugs producing these effects:

1. *Increase release (amphetamine)*
2. *Decrease enzymatic breakdown (pargyline)*
3. *Block pre-synaptic re-uptake (imipramine)*
4. *Stimulate post-synaptic receptors (apomorphine)*

animal performs the specified response, it receives brain stimulation which causes the release of various transmitters. We could therefore say that the "neurochemical purpose" of the self-stimulation response is to facilitate transmitter release. When an animal is given a drug such as amphetamine, one of its effects is to cause each action potential impulse to liberate more transmitter. Consequently, it is to be expected that a release-facilitator such as amphetamine would increase reward. The situation is different in the case of the other three types of transmitter facilitating agents. They also facilitate transmission but the facilitation is produced even if the subject does nothing at all. If transmission is facilitated without the animal having to make any effort, it is unlikely to work for brain stimulation. Under these circumstances, reduced vigour of the instrumental response might be expected, and in fact appears to occur with all of the drugs.

The neurochemical 'purpose' of a self-stimulation response is to alter transmitter release. When this is done pharmacologically in a way that is independent of the self-stimulation response, the response becomes superfluous and its vigour is reduced.

At this stage it is premature to characterize brain stimulation reward as being due to the activation of any one transmitter system. Intuitively, it seems more likely that there are many different types of reward, each with neurochemical profiles reflecting the differential contribution of a number of transmitter systems. We shall see in Chapter 11 that this view is in accord with recent findings from research on the biochemistry of depression. As in the case of self-stimulation, psychiatric depression was originally viewed as reflecting the activity of one neurotransmitter system. Recently, however, and again as with self-stimulation, depression has been characterized as a biochemically diverse phenomenon with a correspondingly diverse group of appropriate treatments.

Questions

1 Explain why a post-synaptic receptor stimulant and a receptor antagonist can both inhibit self-stimulation.
2 How would you go about determining if a rat is really "having fun" while self-stimulating?
3 Consider what it is about rewarding brain stimulation that becomes aversive.
4 Why is it that so few drugs really enhance self-stimulation?

Further Readings

Fibiger, H.C. Drugs and reinforcement mechanisms: A critical review. *Annual Review of Pharmacology and Toxicology*, 1978, **18**, 37–56.
Gallistel, C.R. Self-stimulation: The neurophysiology of reward and motivation. In J.A. Deutsch (Ed.) *The Physiological Basis of Memory*. New York, Academic Press. 1973.

Mogenson, G. and Cioe, J. Central reinforcement — a bridge between brain function and behavior. *In* W.K. Honig and J.E.R. Staddon (Eds) *Handbook of Operant Behavior*. Englewood Cliffs, N.J., Prentice-Hall. 1977.

Valenstein, E.S. Problems of measurement and interpretation with reinforcing brain stimulation. *Psychological Review*, 1964, **71**, 415–437.

Wauquier, A. and Rolls, E.T. (Eds) *Brain-Stimulation Reward*. Amsterdam, North Holland. 1976.

9

Emotions, Sex and Aggression

9.1 Introduction

Emotions, sex and aggression are core elements in any comprehensive analysis of behaviour. Although the neurosciences can potentially make major contributions to the understanding of emotions, sex and aggression progress has been greatly hindered by conceptual and terminological problems. For example, most observers would readily agree on what constitutes seeing, hearing, sleeping, eating, drinking and even learning. In contrast, there are vast differences in opinion about what should be included in (and excluded from) definitions of emotions, sex and aggression.

These terms are used to cover such a broad range of events that their explanatory utility is frequently overstrained. For example, just because fear and anger would both be classed as emotions, there is little reason to expect them to have a similar physiological basis. In other words, it may be quite unreasonable to expect to find something as vague as an emotion system in the brain. Similarly, there is little reason to believe that behaviour as diverse as courtship, copulation and maternal care would have a common physiology, even though they may all be considered to be sexual. Very much the same arguments can be made concerning the diverse forms of aggression.

However, in spite of the great diversity among and within the categories of emotions, sex and aggression there are three physiological systems which play a major role in all of them. These categories form a natural trio because of their common dependence on the autonomic nervous system, the endocrine system and the limbic system of the brain. Along with the skeletal motor system, the autonomic and endocrine systems are the major output systems of the brain. The limbic system may be thought of as the major brain area which controls and integrates the activities of the autonomic and endocrine systems.

9.2 Theories of emotion

The first systematic theory of emotions was developed in the late 19th century by William James and Carl Lange. The James–Lange theory is interesting because it is at odds with traditional views gathered from informal impressions of our emotional experience. It also draws attention to the importance of feedback from peripheral effectors to the brain.

Over the past 100 years or so, the neurosciences have shifted towards emphasizing the pre-eminence of the central nervous system in the determination of behaviour, while relegating the peripheral nervous system to a position of functional insignificance. A more recent trend is to recognize the interactions between the two systems. After all, a disembodied brain or a brainless body are equally ineffective.

Conventional thinking about a typical emotional situation is exemplified as follows. On encountering a menacing situation we become frightened. Because we are frightened, our hearts race, and if we are extremely frightened our hair may stand on end. These and numerous other peripheral sensations result from the activation of the sympathetic division of the autonomic nervous system. In other words, the traditional view is that sympathetic arousal occurs because we are frightened. James and Lange reversed this position and reasoned that we are frightened because of the occurrence of the sympathetic arousal; that is, fear is nothing more than the perception of our autonomic nervous systems over-reacting.

The James–Lange theory has been criticized on a number of grounds by the proponents of the Cannon–Bard theory. However, the criticisms have generally proved irrelevant. Perhaps the strongest criticism made of the peripheralist James–Lange theory by the Cannon–Bard school was that individuals with severed peripheral neural connections to the brain, as occurs in quadriplegia, still experience emotions. Recent study has provided evidence that even this criticism may not be entirely valid. For example, on closer examination quadriplegics do appear to experience attenuated emotions in some situations. They report feeling "as if" they were afraid or angry.

The possibility exists that the residual emotions of quadriplegics reflect a learned and primarily verbal response acquired before the spinal break. This view is supported by studies

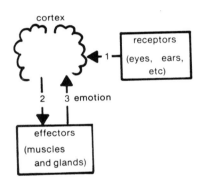

Illustration of the James-Lange peripheral theory of emotions. The numbers on the arrows indicate the proposed sequence of events.

indicating that various laboratory animals that have undergone surgical removal of the sympathetic division of the autonomic nervous system show a predictable deficit in emotional situations. Sympathectomized animals experience little difficulty in performing a shock-avoidance task learned before the sympathectomy. However, if the sympathectomy is performed before the shock-avoidance training, they show little, if any, learning.

Cannon and Bard developed the first neural theory of emotions. They speculated that emotionally relevant sensory messages pass through the thalamus to the cortex where they break the inhibitory influence that the cortex exerts on the thalamus. Once released from inhibition, the thalamus activates the sympathetic component of the autonomic nervous system. The resulting physiological responses occur with, but are not essential to, the emotion. Emotions result from the message from the thalamus as it is released from cortical inhibition.

Among the more remarkable aspects of this theory are its longevity and the fact that it was not experimentally based but was purely speculative. Their hypothetical optic-thalamo-cortical circuit was perhaps the first comprehensive neural "system" proposed to account for a complex behaviour. As such it stands as the immediate ideological precursor to the limbic system, the circuit most widely believed by neuroscientists to be the fundamental neural substrate of emotions (9.10).

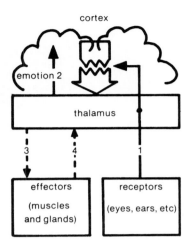

Illustration of the Cannon-Bard central theory of emotions. Essential links appear as solid lines, whereas the non-essential links are dashed. The numbers on the arrows indicate the proposed sequence of events. In this case the emotion is the message sent to the cortex from the thalamus as it is released from chronic cortical inhibition.

9.3 Emotions and the autonomic nervous system

One of the fundamental problems with emotions is the need to infer them from behaviour. Humans' verbal reports of their own emotional states are notoriously unreliable, and laboratory animals, while they may have little reason to be deceptive, cannot provide verbal reports at all. Consequently, it is essential to have objective indices of emotion. Moreover, it is necessary not only to determine whether a subject is experiencing an emotion, but also to differentiate among the various emotions.

The scientific study of emotions requires objective measures of emotion.

While each of us can normally distinguish when we are happy, sad, afraid, angry, randy or belligerent, the problem is to objectify these subjective states. We can see that there is a semantic or perhaps conceptual problem here. Except at the extremes of emotional experience, we probably never experience only one emotion at a time. Even supposedly opposite emotions such as happy and sad may occur concurrently. Certainly, all of the emotions mentioned above can occur in many different combinations. Consequently, any emotional situation undoubtedly elicits a complex pattern of emotions and, at best, we can only speculate about what might be the dominant emotion. This complexity is reflected in the nature of the physiological correlates of emotions.

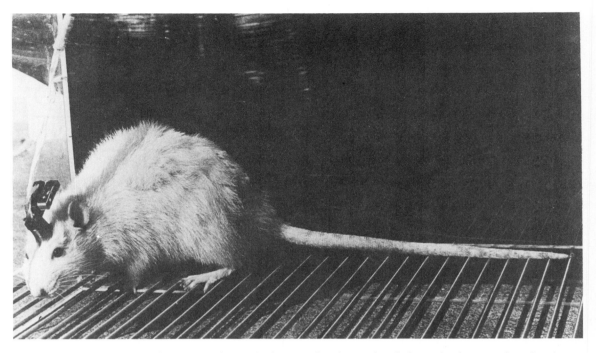

A rat implanted with electrodes for stimulating the brain and with peripheral electrodes for recording the electro-cardiogram. The small device attached to the skull cap assembly is an FM microtransmitter which broadcasts the electro-cardiogram to a nearby polygraph system. This preparation is useful in studying the cardiovascular responses to a wide range of experimental variables.

Emotions involve patterns of responding of the brain, the muscles, and the autonomic and endocrine systems.

During emotional experiences, various components of the central, peripheral and autonomic nervous systems, as well as the endocrine system, are activated. These appear in our folk wisdom as one's heart skipping a beat, heavy breathing, flushed skin, sweaty palms, and a host of other physiological events associated with emotion. Many autonomic responses, such as heart rate, blood pressure, respiration rate and skin conductivity, may be measured by a polygraph system. This research approach is called *psychophysiology*.

A classic psychophysiological investigation of emotions was Ax's attempt to differentiate fear and anger. Ax claimed that of 14 indices of autonomic function, 7 distinguished fear from anger. An interesting extension of this psychophysiological research is the use of the polygraph as a "lie-detector". This application of psychophysiology is based on the largely untested assumption that while we can lie verbally, our autonomic nervous systems are not capable of such deceit.

Perhaps the most important observation made by Ax was the fact that there were marked individual differences in the autonomic responses to emotional situations. Each person seems to have rather idiosyncratic ways of responding to emotions, suggesting that different patterns of autonomic responses may be learned. These findings may explain the dramatically different reactions to stress of various individuals. For example, in response to stress some people develop cardiovascular problems, some develop gastric ulcers, some develop migraine headaches, some become asthmatic, some develop a stutter or a tic, whereas a few appear to emerge unscathed.

The above physiological disorders (and many more) that are caused or precipitated by stress are termed *psychosomatic*. Diseases that are purely biological in origin may be exacerbated by psychosomatic factors. While there is substantial disagreement on the proportion of non-psychiatric medical problems having a major psychosomatic component, estimates range from 30–70%. These figures suggest the need for, and importance of, further research in this area.

Following the argument of Cannon, the autonomic aspects of emotions are usually viewed as terminal physiological output. Since Cannon viewed the responses as rather incidental, and certainly of no causal significance to emotions, their consideration could have ended here. However, recent investigations have shown an important bi-directionality of influence.

Rather than being the simple physiological effluvia of the brain, autonomic responses can also act back on the brain and alter its activity. For example, Lacey and others have shown that, within different phases of the cardiac and respiratory cycle, human reaction time varies considerably. It has also been shown that when males were given false feedback of their own heart rate while examining pictures of nudes, the false information had a large effect on their evaluation of the relative attractiveness of the models. Pictures that were accompanied by a falsified high heart rate were usually evaluated as being more attractive. The evaluations persisted even when the subjects were told that they had been deceived. Clearly, the way our bodies respond influences the activity of the central nervous system.

Skeletal, autonomic and endocrine activity can all modify the activity of the brain.

9.4 The endocrine system

In Chapter 1 we noted that ultimately the organism has only two types of output or effector responses. One involves the contraction of muscles, the other the secretion of glands. There are two types of glands, exocrine and endocrine. The exocrine glands, such as the salivary and tear glands, deliver their secretions through ducts into sites outside the bloodstream. As the exocrine glands have little effect on behaviour they will not be considered further here. The endocrine glands are ductless glands which secrete *hormones* directly into the bloodstream. The hormones are distributed by the bloodstream to "targets" throughout the body. Some hormones have very specific targets (i.e. another endocrine gland), whereas other hormones are very nonspecific and affect cells all over the body. The endocrine

The endocrine system is a chemical communication system which acts in parallel to the nervous system.

system may be thought of as a relatively slow-acting chemical communication system which acts parallel to, and in concert with, the nervous system. Changes in endocrine function are an important element in emotions, sex and aggression.

Hormones fall into three main chemical classes: amines, peptides, and steroids. Since amines and peptides are also major classes of neurotransmitter, it should come as no surprise that the same chemical can act between cells as a neurotransmitter or in the bloodstream as a hormone. However, apart from the difference in the way in which they reach their target, neurotransmitters and hormones affect their targets in different ways. Neurotransmitters diffuse across the synaptic gap where they alter the electrical state of the postsynaptic cell. In contrast, hormones rarely initiate chemical reactions. They more typically modulate the rates of ongoing reactions. Hormones could be thought of as physiological catalysts except that, in marked contrast to catalysts, hormones are consumed by the reactions whose rates they alter.

Hormones are the message units of the endocrine system.

A joint neurotransmitter–hormonal role was first documented for noradrenalin. However, recent evidence suggests that many of the peptide hormones in particular may also serve as neurotransmitters. In some cases the peptides appear to produce effects on neurotransmission that have a much longer latency and duration than conventional neurotransmitters. The rather slow temporal course of their effects has led to their being called *neuromodulators*. It is likely that some substances may serve as hormones, neurotransmitters and neuromodulators.

Some substances act both as neurotransmitters and hormones.

The most important gland in the endocrine system is the *pituitary* or *hypophysis*. The pituitary, which dangles from the base of the brain just above the roof of your mouth, is an interface between the brain and the endocrine system. In response to specific releasing factors produced in the hypothalamus and transported to it by the local circulation, the anterior pituitary (or adenohypophysis) releases various hormones into the general circulation. These anterior pituitary hormones generally exert their effect by altering the hormonal secretion of the other endocrine glands. For example, the hypothalamus secretes *thyrotrophin releasing factor,* which travels through the pituitary portal blood vessels to the anterior pituitary. The thyrotrophin releasing factor causes the anterior pituitary to secrete *thyrotrophin* into the general circulation. The thyrotrophin is transported by the blood to the thyroid gland where it stimulates the release of *thyroxine*. It is the thyroxine which produces the ultimate effect exerted by the thyroid gland.

Some primary hormones (oxytocin and vasopressin) are also synthesized in the hypothalamus and then transported to the posterior pituitary where they are stored for later use. Because these hormones are transported along nerve axons to their storage site, the posterior pituitary is also called the *neurohypophysis*.

Thus hormonal secretion often involves a rather complex sequence of releasing factors (such as thyrotrophin releasing factor) and intermediary hormones (such as thyrotrophin) which ultimately results in the secretion of a primary hormone (such as thyroxine). The distinctions between releasing factors, intermediary hormones and primary hormones are rather arbitrary. Both releasing factors and intermediary hormones may also in some cases act as primary hormones or neurotransmitters, or as both.

The table below alphabetically lists the major endocrine glands, some of their hormones and the general regulatory spheres in which they operate. This table is incomplete in several respects. More hormones could have been added and vastly greater breadth and precision of hormonal effects could have been achieved. However, such breadth and precision is incompatible with brevity.

GLAND	TYPICAL HORMONE(S)	REGULATORY FUNCTION
adenohypophysis (*see* pituitary, anterior)		
adrenal cortex	cortisol	energy utilization, anti-inflammation
	aldosterone	electrolyte balance
adrenal medulla	adrenalin	energy utilization, cardiovascular function
	noradrenalin	energy utilization, cardiovascular function
gastrointestinal tract	cholecystokinin	gall bladder contractions
kidney	angiotensin II	electrolyte balance
neurohypophysis (*see* pituitary, posterior)		
ovary	oestradiol	sex characteristics and behaviour
pancreas	insulin	blood glucose lowering, increases fat synthesis
	glucagon	blood glucose raising, increases fat breakdown
parathyroid	parathormone	blood electrolyte balance

GLAND	TYPICAL HORMONE(S)	REGULATORY FUNCTION
pituitary anterior	adrenocorticotrophin	releases adrenal steroids
	follicle stimulating hormone	growth of ovarian follicles and sperm development
	lutenizing hormone	ovulation and secretion of androgens from the testes
	prolactin	milk secretion
	somatotrophin (growth hormone)	growth
	thyrotrophin	stimulates thyroid
posterior	oxytocin	delivery of foetus and milk secretion
	vasopressin (antidiuretic hormone)	fluid retention
testes	testosterone	male sex characteristics and behaviour
thymus	lymphocytes	immunological reactions
thyroid	thyroxine	energy utilization, differentiation during development

9.5 The endocrinology of stress

In addition to autonomic responses to emotional situations, there is a powerful endocrine reaction which is a major contributor to the overall physiological response pattern. Cannon claimed that during emergency situations the adrenal medulla secretes adrenalin and noradrenalin into the blood stream. These hormones, along with the activation of the sympathetic division of the autonomic nervous system, prepare the organism for a massive and immediate expenditure of energy. The well-worn phrase describing this kind of physiological response is the "fight or flight" reaction. This concept was further developed by Hans Selye, who maintained that during stress virtually the entire endocrine system is activated in a monolithic and non-specific manner. He called it the "general adaptation syndrome".

However, the endocrine response to stress is neither general nor is it always adaptive. Mason, Levine and others have provided evidence suggesting that, as is the case with autonomic responses, endocrine responses to stress are best described as patterns and not as monolithic responses. A non-specific endocrine response would have little adaptive value, since different types of stress require different endocrine responses.

Consider, for example, two different types of thermal stress — extreme cold and extreme heat. To simplify the discussion, we shall consider only the heat-producing hormone thyroxine. Thyroxine secretion would be adaptive to cold stress but mal-adaptive to heat stress. Thus, thyroxine secretion to these two stresses is respectively increased and decreased. To other non-thermal stresses, thyroxine secretion may not change at all.

Schachter has demonstrated a feedback influence of endocrine responses on emotional behaviour. He injected volunteers with adrenalin to simulate artificial activation of the adrenal medulla. Since adrenalin does not cross the blood–brain barrier, any effects it produces should be confined to the periphery. He found that, when paired with a stooge who acted either playful or hostile, the adrenalin-injected subjects showed an enhancement in either emotion. In contrast, saline-injected control subjects showed no change in emotions. This indicates that the peripheral activation acted back on the central nervous system to amplify whatever emotion was currently been elicited by the environment.

Although the diverse forms of stress have traditionally been considered to be equivalent, recent experiments have shown that stress is physiologically and behaviourally far more complex than was believed even a few years ago. Although Mason, Levine and others have shown that different types of stress produce different patterns of endocrine responses, it was widely believed that these were simply different reflections of a common underlying stress mechanism.

Some of the best evidence against the existence of a single stress mechanism comes from studies of *stress-induced analgesia*. Stress produced by electric foot shock, swimming in cold water, vigorous running and metabolic poisons produces an analgesia much like that produced by morphine. Since morphine has striking effects on brain endorphins, it appeared that stress might also trigger endorphin release. These endogenous opiate-like compounds were even invoked to explain "joggers high", which is a feeling of euphoria reported by some long-distance runners.

A further similarity between stress-induced and morphine analgesia is the tolerance that develops to either one of them. Stress and morphine injections become progressively less effective when repeatedly administered. If there is a common mechanism underlying stress-induced and morphine analgesia, then subjects who have become tolerant to either stress or morphine should also show tolerance to the other, even though they have never experienced it. This phenomenon, which is called *cross-tolerance*,

Different types of stress produce different endocrine responses.

Expectations can substantially modify the effects of many physiological variables.

Acute stress can produce analgesia.

does occur between the stressful metabolic poison 2-deoxy-D-glucose and morphine. There is also cross-tolerance between 2-deoxy-D-glucose and cold-water swimming. However, there is no cross-tolerance between cold-water swimming and morphine. These findings suggest that, even though the two stressors (2-deoxy-D-glucose and cold-water swimming) produce an apparently identical analgesic effect, their underlying neurochemistry is obviously quite different.

Further differentiation of the neurochemical events underlying different stressors has been produced by experiments with the opiate antagonist *naloxone*. Naloxone can block the analgesia produced by morphine, enkephalins, endorphins and acupuncture. However, naloxone does not block the analgesia produced by either 2-deoxy-D-glucose or cold-water swimming. These findings suggest that at least some stressors produce their analgesic effects through non-opiate related mechanisms. Perhaps related to this is the report that naloxone does not antagonize the self-induced analgesia of entertainers who lie on beds of nails.

Stress-induced analgesia appears to involve both opiate-related and non-opiate-related systems in the brain.

It is now known that the endocrine response to stress is highly dependent on psychological factors. For example, electric foot shock increases the output of adrenal steroids and causes an acute depletion of hypothamic noradrenalin. However, the physiological changes to the anticipation of foot shock may be greater than to the actual shock itself. These findings indicate that the expectation of an aversive event may be more stressful than the aversive event itself. Thus principles of learning and conditioning can vastly extend the time scale of the endocrine (and probably autonomic) consequences of stress.

The above considerations suggest that both the physiological and behavioural responses to stress may be modified by learning. These modifications are sometimes adaptive, but under certain circumstances they can be strikingly maladaptive. For example, if rats that have been trained to escape foot shock are given large amounts of inescapable shock, a maladaptive change in behaviour results. When the shock is once again made escapable, the rats no longer attempt to escape it. As a result, they expose themselves to large amounts of stressful shock even though they can easily escape it. This phenomenon, which is called *learned helplessness*, is highly reminiscent of some types of human psychiatric dysfunction. Weiss and his colleagues have conducted a number of experiments suggesting that learned helplessness involves a long-term dysfunction in noradrenergic neurons.

Chronic stress can produce chronic behavioural and physiological deficits.

In conclusion, we can see there are some marked similarities in the way our autonomic nervous system and endocrine system respond to emotional or stressful situations. Historically, both were said to be generally activated by stress. However, any appearance of general physiological activation probably indicates that we have not looked carefully. Closer examination reveals complex, patterned autonomic and endocrine responses that probably reflect a high degree of learning.

9.6 Sexual behaviour

As was the case with emotions, the definition of sexual behaviour is a matter of dispute. Whereas most people would agree on definitions of eating, drinking, sweating and shivering, there is a bewildering range of what experts would classify as constituting sexual behaviour. At one extreme is the position that sex simply involves the combination of genetic material between two cells. At the other extreme is the position developed by Sigmund Freud. He claimed that sexual drive was the universal motivating force. According to Freud all behaviour could be considered sexual, and indeed, the more non-sexual any behaviour appears, the more it must be sex-related in reality. Thus, at one extreme sex is defined as including almost nothing, whereas at the other extreme it is defined as including almost everything.

Even when the extremes are avoided, problems of definition still remain. For example, some texts equate sexual behaviour with reproduction and go on to point out the enormous differences between humans and even our closest primate relatives.

Since much human sexual behaviour is not concerned with, indeed may in fact be actively concerned with avoiding, reprodution, it seems that some of the apparent differences may reflect the fact that experimenters tend to stress different aspects of behaviour in the various species studied. Human sexuality is usually thought to include a wide spectrum of social and emotional factors of which copulation and reproduction may be relatively minor components.

There is an unfortunate tendency to equate sex with reproduction. This seriously oversimplifies both human and animal sexual behaviour.

Comparable events in other animals are generally given little attention. However, even non-primates such as dogs or cats, upon close observation, are seen to display large individual differences in sexual behaviour and a dependence upon what might be called "psychological" factors. Many non-human species show preferences for certain partners and, like humans, they are aroused by stimulus novelty. A male rat that is apparently sexually satiated after repeated copulation with one female will show increased activity if a new female is introduced.

9.7 Sex hormones and development

The main sources of primary sex hormones are the gonads and pituitary gland. The gonads are the ovaries in the female and the testes in the male. The principal hormones secreted by the ovaries are oestrogen and progesterone. The testes secrete two types of hormones called androgens, testosterone and andro-

The gonads in the male are called testes. Those in the female are called ovaries.

stenedione. Both sexes secrete all of the sex hormones but females secrete more oestrogen and progesterone, and the males more androgens. It is an oversimplification to speak of these as being female or male hormones.

Traditionally it has been thought that sex hormones function mainly to promote sexual maturity and to facilitate sexual behaviour in the adult. However, hormones exert a far broader influence on both prenatal and postnatal development than had previously been suspected. Prenatal injections of the androgen testosterone into the mother of a genetically female monkey produce a striking masculinization in the physiology of the offspring. Further, in a number of social situations the offspring show behaviour that is more typical of males than females.

After birth, two additional methods may be used in manipulating the hormonal environment. In addition to injecting hormones, the gonads can be transplanted or removed. Removal of the ovaries in the female or the testes in the male is called castration. Castration in males, particularly shortly after birth, greatly increases the likelihood of that individual showing feminine behaviour, and similarly decreases the likelihood of male behaviour. The administration of oestrogens during the development of a castrated male does not increase the feminization of the male.

Castration feminizes males, but it does not masculinize females.

Castration in young females delays the development of female characteristics, but it does not result in the appearance of masculine characteristics. Only when castrated young females are also treated with testosterone does a distinct masculinization take place. These results generally indicate that early castration in either sex results in essentially feminine physiological development and behaviour. Testosterone will masculinize castrates of either sex.

We can conclude that, both physiologically and behaviourally, organisms of both sexes have a built-in female bias. The androgen testosterone functions to superimpose a masculine structure on what is basically a feminine foundation. In this context, the other androgen, androstenedione, occupies a unique position. Androstenedione administration to castrates of either sex facilitates the appearance of homosexual behaviour in addition to heterosexual behaviour. In other words, androstenedione appears to facilitate the development of bisexual behaviour. The fact that we have sex hormones that could loosely be called female, male and bisexual underscores the absurdity of sexual chauvinism in members of either sex.

9.8 Sex hormones and adult sexual behaviour

The above discussion focused on the hormonal regulation of physiological and behavioural development. Hormones also play an important role in adult sexual behaviour. It is interesting to note that the dichotomy in terms of sexual performance between mature and immature individuals in a number of species has been overstated. For example, immature males and females when treated with appropriate hormones will show essentially "normal" adult copulatory behaviour, suggesting that the physiological mechanisms for copulation are developed well before that behaviour appears. All that is required is an appropriate hormone trigger. Consequently, the sexual developmental lag reflects the relatively slow development of underlying hormonal mechanisms.

The importance of hormones in sex-related physiological characteristics and behaviour is often stressed at the expense of another important determining factor, that of experience or learning. While hormonal changes may be said to "cause" sexual behaviour, behaviour itself may influence hormonal changes. Thus the effects of many hormonal changes will depend on the current behavioural state of the organism, and on its previous history.

It is sometimes forgotten that, while hormones alter behaviour, behaviour also alters hormonal activity.

An excellent example of experience–hormone interactions is provided by the effects of castration on copulation in male cats. If a virgin male is castrated, it will probably never copulate with a female, even if given testosterone "replacement therapy". In contrast, the sexual behaviour of an old, experienced cat will be surprisingly little affected by castration. If a decline in sexual activity occurs, it is typically minor and may take a long time to appear at all. Further, if there is any decline in sexual performance, testosterone replacement therapy will immediately restore it to pre-castration levels.

The effects of castration on males can be greatly reduced by previous sexual experience.

Similar findings have been reported for castrated male humans. It appears that sexual experience changes the male physiologically and behaviourally so as to render sexual behaviour relatively independent of testosterone. In this respect the human female resembles the male in showing a high degree of hormonal-independence.

Castrated women or women who have gone through menopause, when the cyclic production of sex hormones ceases, report relatively little loss of sexual interest. On the other hand, females of non-human species show complete dependence on hormones. Adult castrates appear to lose interest in copulation, and will actively resist the advances of even the most ardent male. Ovarian transplant or appropriate hormone-replacement therapy is necessary to restore sexual receptivity.

Castration in non-human females invariably completely eliminates copulation.

There is a second point of difference between males and females in the control of sexual behaviour. In females "sexual interest" can be equated with ability to copulate. Males not only have to be interested but they also have to achieve and maintain an erect penis. This suggests that male sexual performance is more likely than the female to be hindered by a variety of sensory or motor deficits. This is supported by experiments in which dogs were subjected to an extensive removal of the cerebral cortex. Females were relatively unaffected, whereas copulation was completely abolished in males. It is argued that the sex difference reflects the higher level of sensorimotor coordination necessary to the male in maintaining an active role in copulation.

9.9 Neural control of sexual behaviour

Hormones are important for the development and maintenance of both the physiological and behavioural aspects of sexual function. Since hormonal secretion is largely regulated by the pituitary, which in turn is regulated by the hypothalamus, it is apparent that the final regulation of sexual functioning is effected in the brain. However, two of the basic motor patterns of male copulation, erection and ejaculation appear to be somewhat independent of the brain.

Spinal damage may actually increase the vigour of some sexual reflexes.

For example, a high spinal break results in *quadriplegia*. Quadriplegics have no neural connections between the brain and skeletal muscle of any parts of the body below the break. Yet male quadriplegics show erection and ejaculation that is unimpaired, and in some cases even better than that of intact males. Besides showing that penile erection and ejaculation are organized at the level of the spinal cord, these results suggest that the brain acts primarily to inhibit the spinal mechanisms. When the inhibition is eliminated, the responses are facilitated. Since quadriplegics also show complete motor paralysis, copulation itself is, of course, seriously impaired.

Nearly every manipulation of the brain interferes with sexual behaviour.

With the above-mentioned exception of the apparent facilitation of male spinal sexual reflexes and one or two other exceptions, nearly any manipulation of the brain interferes with sexual behaviour. The few clear instances of sexual behaviour enhanced by brain manipulations may be restricted to a small number of species.

The generally inhibitory effects of brain lesions, in particular, should not be surprising in light of the preceding discussion on the complex sequence of hormonal and sensorimotor events underlying copulation and other sexual behaviours. A wide range of neural manipulations can disrupt one or more of these components and, consequently, interfere with sexual behaviour. The question to be asked is: "Does the inhibition represent a primary reduction in sexuality or is it instead due to a non-specific interference with motor function?"

An inability to copulate does not necessarily indicate loss of the sexual urge. During an interview shortly before his death, Groucho Marx made a sweeping gesture around his study indicating a large collection of awards and honours. "See those. I'd trade them all for one erection."

Although there are reports of copulation elicited by electrical stimulation of the hypothalamus, the findings may have limited application generally. First, it is a low probability phenomenon occurring in a small percentage of cases. Further, it seems to be restricted to male rats. Other species and sexes may show fragments of the copulation pattern but rarely an organized copulation sequence. Since male rats will also show copulation in response to a mild tail pinch, the copulation induced by brain stimulation may be artifactual.

Another often-cited example of facilitating sexual behaviour is the report by Klüver and Bucy of hypersexuality in cats following extensive lesions of the temporal lobe. The cats were reported to have attempted copulation with inanimate objects such as stuffed dogs or other "inappropriate" objects such as other male cats or the experimenter's glove.

However, recent studies indicate that the conclusion reached by Klüver and Bucy may have been incorrect. First, all the behaviours they considered to indicate hypersexuality are found in cats with intact brains. Klüver and Bucy may not have made adequate pre-operative observations in their cats. Second, some of the apparent hypersexuality may reflect a general disruption in the cats' ability to discriminate appropriate objects or situations. In other words, the cats' attempts at copulating with the experimenter's hand may have been due to their inability to distinguish the inappropriateness of this object, and not to excessive sexuality.

The apparent hypersexuality following temporal lobe damage may be a problem of discrimination not of excessive sex drive.

9.10 The limbic system

The limbic system remains the major point of focus of research into brain mechanisms of emotions, sex and aggression. Various limbic subdivisions, in particular the hypothalamus, exert a major modulating influence on the autonomic and endocrine responses, which are major components of emotions, sex and aggression. The limbic system, in turn, is generally thought to integrate and process messages to and from the sensory areas of the cortex.

The notion of a neural system composed of interconnected components, each of which has a particular emotion-related function, was largely developed by Papez and MacClean. The anatomical term from which the limbic system concept was developed was provided by Broca in the 19th century. The term "limbic" comes from the Latin "limbus" meaning border. Broca defined the "limbic lobe" as a discrete group of structures which form a border between the brain stem and the neocortex. Contemporary use of the term "limbic system" is far broader and less precise than that of Broca.

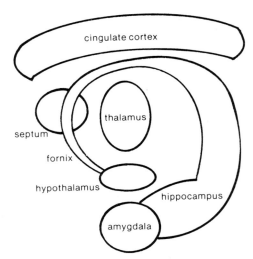

Representation of some of the major components of the human limbic system. The view is from the left side and the brain has been sectioned along its front-to-rear axis.

The limbic system is usually considered to include the limbic lobe as defined by Broca as well as various "associated" subcortical structures. Because of the extensive interconnectivity of brain structures, virtually any part of the brain stem or neocortex could be considered to be associated with, and hence be part of, the limbic system. In the absence of more precise anatomical, physiological or behavioural criteria it is doubtful whether "the limbic system" is a useful term. For the purposes of this work we will define the limbic system as shown in the accompanying illustration.

The following discussion indicates that many structures traditionally considered as belonging to the limbic system are, indeed, involved in emotions, sex and aggression. However, for several reasons we remain sceptical about the overall usefulness of the limbic system concept. First, in many cases it is still not clear whether the effects of various limbic manipulations represent primary changes in behaviour or are instead secondary changes which are due to non-specific disruption of behaviour. Second, many of the changes appear to be very situational and species-specific. Third, we will see below (9.21) that many diseases of the human limbic system produce no obvious changes in emotions, sex and aggression. More so than with many areas of neuroscience research, this area is plagued with the problem of distinguishing fact from artifact.

These cautions should not be interpreted as suggesting that the numerous changes in behaviour produced by limbic system manipulations are neither meaningful nor interesting. The point of this critical discussion is that our current basic knowledge of limbic system function is so limited that it does not yet warrant clinical application (see 9.22).

9.11 Aggression

As is the case with emotions and sex, aggression is clearly not a unitary category of behaviour and, as such, will not submit to a unitary physiological explanation. There are many different kinds of aggression, for example predatory, affective, shock-induced, isolation-induced, etc. It appears that the peripheral physiology and brain involvement in each of these diverse behaviours is different.

We shall first consider basic research on aggression in laboratory animals and then examine human aggression and the use of psychosurgery.

9.12 The hypothalamus and aggression

The hypothalamus may be thought of as the anatomical axis about which the other major limbic areas (septum, amygdala, hippocampus, and neocortex) are organized. Physiologically, its demonstrated importance to both endocrine and autonomic functions indicates its probable involvement in emotions, sex and aggression. Cannon postulated the idea some 50 years ago, and there is now considerable supporting evidence.

Some of the most interesting experiments in this area have been conducted by Flynn and associates at Yale University. Flynn found that electrical stimulation of the lateral hypothalamus in cats evoked a deliberate, stealthy and well-organized form of predatory aggression which he called "quiet stalking attack". In contrast, medial hypothalamic stimulation evoked an explosive, hissing, spitting and clawing type of predation called "affective attack". In each case the objective of the attack was the same – killing the rat. However, this was virtually the only similarity between the two types of aggression.

Electrical stimulation of the lateral hypothalamus in cats produces 'quiet stalking attack'.

Electrical stimulation of the medial hypothalamus in cats produces 'affective (enraged) attack'.

Results from experiments in which the two hypothalamic components have been lesioned are not in complete accordance with the stimulation results. For example, destruction of the lateral hypothalamus appears to reduce aggressiveness (along with the vigour of almost every other behaviour). On the other hand, a cat with a lateral hypothalamic lesion on only one side of the brain will show great interest in, and possibly attack, a rat in one half of its visual field, while completely ignoring a rat in the other half of its visual field. The results argue against the loss of predatory aggression as being a generalized disturbance. So, with respect to the involvement of the lateral hypothalamus in predatory aggression, the lateral hypothalamic stimulation and lesion results are complementary.

The case with respect to medial hypothalamic involvement in aggression is not as clear. Since stimulation of the medial hypothalamus produces affective attack, it would be reasonable to expect that lesions of the medial hypothalamus would inhibit the same behaviour. However, medial hypothalamic lesions almost universally produce a marked increase in most forms of aggression. This type of paradoxical result in the study of emotionality often characterizes experimental manipulations of limbic function.

9.13 The septum and aggression

Septal involvement in aggression is one of the more coherent aspects of research on emotion. Large septal lesions produce a large, but transient increase in viciousness and emotionality. If the lesions are restricted to the medial septum, they produce docility and decreased emotionality. As is the case with the medial hypothalamus, electric stimulation of the septum generally produces effects that are parallel to, and not complementary with, those produced by lesions.

Large septal lesions frequently produce exaggerated emotional responses.

Lateral septal stimulation increases emotionality and aggressiveness, whereas medial septal stimulation either decreases or has no effect on these responses. However, whereas the effects of hypothalamic stimulation occur only during stimulation, the effects of septal stimulation appear primarily after stimulation. It suggests that the latter effects may represent some sort of seizure-like after-effect. The results further suggest that a variety of apparent increases in emotionality and aggression may be due to seizure activity secondary to a particular brain manipulation. In other words, the principal anatomical focus of a given brain manipulation may be incidental to, and remote from, the part of the brain being investigated.

9.14 The amygdala and aggression

Perhaps the main pillar supporting the traditional view of the limbic system as the fundamental neural substrate of emotion is the report of Klüver and Bucy concerning the effects on emotional behaviour of removing the amygdala. The main features of the Klüver–Bucy syndrome are docility, orality and hypersexuality. Savage animals, such as the lynx, became placid and easy to handle after the operation. They also showed a rather indiscriminate mouthing of objects, including sharp nails and lit matches. The reported hypersexuality is of less interest since later experiments have indicated that probably it did not represent hypersexuality at all. Instead, it may reflect that the experimenters failed to measure pre-operative sexual behaviour adequately (see 9.9).

Since such findings constitute a large part of the experimental basis for the surgical control of human violence, it is remarkable that the large amount of contrary experimental evidence is generally ignored. For example, Bard and Mountcastle demonstrated that amygdalectomy greatly increased the expression of rage. The fact that amygdalectomy may also produce excessive orality and inappropriate sexual behaviour suggests that the taming effect may simply reflect a general state of disorientation and confusion. Inconclusive and contradictory evidence such as this hardly constitutes a reasonable basis for the destruction of human brain tissue to control aggression.

The effects of temporal lobe lesions on emotionality are so variable and indiscriminate that their use in controlling human violence has been seriously questioned.

9.15 The frontal lobes

Although the frontal lobes are not generally considered part of the limbic system, they merit consideration in any discussion of the neural basis of emotions. The development of frontal lobe surgery in humans is a classic example of the misunderstanding and consequent misapplication of the results of basic brain research. In 1935 Jacobsen reported that damage to the frontal lobes resulted in the following changes in the behaviour of monkeys — decreased aggression, impaired temporal memory and stereotyped, rigid behaviour patterns. On the basis of the first findings and in apparent ignorance of, or disregard for, the other two, Moniz developed the procedure of prefrontal lobotomy for humans.

Although originally developed as a treatment for aggression, lobotomy and the related procedure of leucotomy were, for a time, used for treating a wide variety of behavioural disorders ranging from schizophrenia to jay-walking. Because the adverse effects of the procedures usually outweigh any positive therapeutic effects, their use is becoming increasingly rare.

9.16 The neurochemistry of aggression

Insight into the neurochemistry of spontaneous aggression has been provided by experiments in which various pharmacological treatments have been used to induce aggression in laboratory animals. These experiments suggest a major excitatory role for the catecholamines noradrenalin (NA) and dopamine (DA). This does not exclude significant roles for other transmitters; however

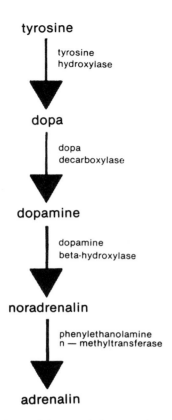

tyrosine

tyrosine hydroxylase

dopa

dopa decarboxylase

dopamine

dopamine beta-hydroxylase

noradrenalin

phenylethanolamine n — methyltransferase

adrenalin

Synthesis of the catecholamine neurotransmitters (dopamine, noradrenalin, adrenalin) from their precursor amino acid tyrosine. The tyrosine is obtained from the digestion of proteins and is transported to the brain via the bloodstream. The enzymes catalysing each reaction are also included.

Human violence is only rarely associated with brain dysfunction.

the role of the catecholamines is presently the best understood.

NA and DA may be sequentially synthesized from DOPA. Since peripherally administered DOPA crosses the blood–brain barrier, it produces an increase in the availability of both NA and DA in the brain. The effect may be further increased by inhibiting monoamine oxidase (MAO), the enzyme that breaks down NA and DA. The administration of DOPA plus a MAO inhibitor causes spontaneous aggression. Further evidence for the catecholaminergic theory of spontaneous aggression is provided by the increase in aggression produced by the catecholamine-liberating drug amphetamine.

Research into the relative importance of the two catecholamines (DA and NA) has provided equivocal results. If the enzyme which converts DA to NA (dopamine-beta-hydroxylase) is inhibited by the drug disulfiram, then any effects of DOPA administration will be due primarily to its increasing the availability of DA. In cats, disulfiram eliminates DOPA-induced aggression, whereas in rodents some reports show a similar reduction but others show no effect. The conflicting results could reflect differences in evaluating and quantifying spontaneous aggression, or they may also indicate a fundamental species difference.

A reduction in aggression (or in any other behaviour) may not necessarily reflect a primary effect, but could instead be secondary to general disturbances in sensory or motor processes. We have seen that the issue of differentiating specific behavioural effects from general changes in activity–reactivity remains a continuing problem in neuroscience research.

9.17 Human violence

We shall consider here the biological basis of human violence and the special case of psychosurgery to control violence. We should first note that violence is neither necessarily pathological nor the expression of our genetic make-up. We live in a world of violence. The aggressive individual gets promoted first, gets movie tickets first, is served first at the bar. The point of these examples is that about 99.9% of violence is not considered evidence of an underlying pathology.

That oscillations of violence occasionally reach alarming proportions is only to be expected. In a society that so conspicuously rewards most forms of violence, to attribute some media-worthy incidents to a brain pathology is premature. Violence is a behavioural problem and its control will ultimately be at the behavioural level. Neurosurgery is appropriate only when there is clear evidence of a neuropathology. Neuropathology is only infrequently associated with human violence. This is reflected in the general lack of success of the surgical treatment of aggression.

9.18 The genetics of human violence

If human violence had a significant genetic component one would expect it to "run in families". Further, there should be a high rate of concordance for twins, especially monozygotic twins. However, the methodological difficulties in separating genetic from environmental effects are so formidable that the genetic studies of violence are now given little credence.

Another line of evidence which is suggestive of a genetic contribution to violence concerns the incidence of acts of violence in males with atypical chromosomes. In contrast with the normal XY chromosome pattern, some males have either an extra X (XXY) or Y (XYY) chromosome. Both patterns have been linked with crimes of violence.

In 1965 a team of British researchers identified, in a prison hospital population, a group of symptoms that were strongly associated with the unusual XYY chromosome configuration. While the XYY pattern occurs with a frequency of approximately 0.1% in the general population, it was claimed to occur 30 times more frequently among the inmates. Further, the XYY individuals were much taller than the others. Since the authors could identify no family circumstances that would produce the criminal behaviour, it was concluded that the extra Y chromosome produced both increased height and an increased tendency to be violent. Other investigations have reported a similar picture of a tall, violent man associated with an extra X chromosome (XXY) — the Klinefelter syndrome.

Evaluation of these results is complicated by a number of methodological problems. For example, it is not appropriate to compare XYY or XXY incidence in imprisoned males with that in the general population. For a comparison to be meaningful it would require a control group of non-imprisoned males matched closely for age, ethnic group, social class, drug use, and so on. This has not yet been done. Further, the laboratory procedures used for detecting chromosomal abnormalities vary widely, and while some are reliable, others are not. Since the overall incidence of the chromosomal abnormalities is low, a small error factor in the chromosome analyses could obscure or accentuate any real differences. Finally, many people with the chromosome patterns (XXY, XYY) lead perfectly normal lives. These considerations suggest that, at best, the chromosomal abnormalities may provide a slight genetic bias towards violence. Once again it appears that the major determinants of violence are environmental.

The data associating male chromosomal abnormalities with violence are, at best, equivocal.

9.19 Epilepsy and violence

Epilepsy is characterized by episodes of uncontrolled electrical "storms" both in cortical and subcortical areas. They may result in similarly uncontrolled episodes of motor dysfunction that are called *epileptic seizures*. Since these storms of electrical–behavioural dysfunction often originate in the limbic cortex (temporal lobe), there has been considerable effort to associate them with episodic fits of violence. For example, Mark and Ervin reported that epilepsy was ten times more common in the prison population. In contrast, Rodin observed 57 epileptics during seizure and found no cases of increased aggressiveness either during or after the seizure. In a larger study which involved examining case histories and interviewing of 700 epileptics, Rodin found no higher incidence of violence than in the general population. While the issue is by no means closed, it is apparent that considerable methodological improvements are necessary if further research is to provide us with concrete findings.

9.20 Disease-induced brain lesions and violence

An important line of investigation into brain mechanisms of behaviour in humans is to observe the changes in behaviour produced by brain tumours and other disease states. One of the first correlations between a brain abnormality and abnormal emotional behaviour was made by Papez. He observed the intense emotional and convulsive symptoms of rabies and noted that rabies caused damage to the hippocampus. The use of this correlation to support the overall limbic–emotional system hypothesis is somewhat peculiar, since hippocampal lesions in laboratory animals (which provide the bulk of the evidence of the hypothesis) generally produce no obvious changes in emotionality. As described earlier, the limbic area most clearly implicated in emotions is the hypothalamus. The autopsy data collected by Von Economo following the encephalitis lethargica (sleeping sickness) plague of 1920, indicated that damage to the hypothalamus was often associated with hyperactivity and aggression.

Many diseases damage the limbic system, yet they produce no changes in emotionality.

There have since been many investigations of the emotional changes following disease-induced damage to the hippocampus and hypothalamus in humans. Kernicterus, herpes encephalitis, Wernicke syndrome and Boeck sarcoid all produce extensive limbic damage with no noticeable changes in emotionality. These results reinforce the opinion that damage to the limbic system in humans is neither a necessary nor sufficient condition to produce changes in emotional behaviour.

9.21 Psychosurgery

Psychosurgery, which is the use of neurosurgery to control behavioural problems, is an extremely controversial mode of therapy. At one end of the spectrum are advocates of psychosurgery, such as Mark and Ervin, who have attempted to attribute most violence to an underlying brain pathology. Those who oppose psychosurgery may be divided into two groups. The first group is sometimes known as Ethically Concerned Citizens Emphasizing Humanism in Our Medical Operations (ECCE HOMO). These people are not particularly concerned with the effectiveness of psychosurgery. Their main concern is that it might be effective. They see themselves as combatants in a romantic struggle of the human spirit against the surgeon's knife. (This position has been dramatised in works such as *One Flew Over the Cuckoo's Nest*.) They are opposed to behaviour control *per se*, and see the surgical approach as particularly threatening. The dimensions and peculiarities of such contemporary obscurantism have been eloquently described by Skinner in a number of articles, and in books such as *Science and Human Behavior*.

The opponents of psychosurgery see it either as a threat to human liberty or as an ineffective and irreversible form of therapy.

The second group opposes psychosurgery because they believe that it does not work. It is simply "bad medicine". This view has been championed by Elliot Valenstein in his book *Brain Control*. Since it is beyond our scope to consider the entire field of psychosurgery, we shall restrict our discussion to some broad methodological issues. While psychosurgery may be of some therapeutic value, the manner in which it is practised is often open to criticism. There are two main reasons that make psychosurgery appear inadequate in comparison with other medical, even psychiatric, practices.

One reason is that much psychosurgery is frequently based upon a misinterpretation of research with non-human species. For example, whereas Moniz used Jacobsen's results to develop lobotomy, it is unlikely that Jacobsen would have viewed his own results as justifying the application. Similarly, even a cursory examination of the effects of amygdalotomy on animal behaviour is enough to arouse doubts about its general usefulness in controlling human behavioural problems (see 9.14). Psychosurgeons frequently base their procedures upon animal experiments that are years out of date.

A second and equally serious weakness of psychosurgery concerns the evaluation of its outcome. Psychosurgery is almost invariably evaluated by the surgeon or close colleagues with full knowledge of the nature of the operation and the expected (or hoped for) outcome. The experimental surgeon is under great pressure to produce successes. Considering the subjective nature

The highest success rates for both surgical and non-surgical psychiatric treatment are invariably reported by the practitioners themselves.

of many psychiatric judgements, it is not surprising that psycho-surgeons tend to report a high success rate for themselves.

There is a close analogy here with the evaluation of the results of psychoanalysis. Psychoanalysis is almost always judged to be more successful by psychoanalysts than it is by independent observers or the patients themselves. Similarly, psychoanalysis, psychosurgery, and all forms of medical treatment, have a powerful placebo effect. In other words, a positive therapeutic effect may not be due to the therapy as such, but rather to the general air of concern and close attention that accompanies the therapy. The placebo effect is likely to be particularly great with a procedure as massive and dangerous as psychosurgery. Placebo effects, while they are worthwhile and even desirable, should not, however, be confused with a primary therapeutic effect. It is this sort of continuing confusion which permitted a surgical excess like lobotomy to continue as long as it did (see 9.15).

The widely reported and extensively dramatized excesses and abuses of psychosurgery should not be interpreted as indicating that it is a dead issue not worthy of further pursuit. There are well-documented cases where absolutely hopeless, non-functional human beings who have failed to respond to all conventional modes of therapy have been restored to some semblance of normality by surgical treatment. However, it is clear that for real progress to be made we shall require new standards of communication between basic and applied neuro-scientists, as well as improved procedures for evaluating the outcome of treatment.

Questions

1 Define emotions.
2 How would you determine if quadriplegics really experience emotions?
3 Compare and contrast neural and hormonal communication.
4 Discuss the usefulness of the limbic system concept.
5 Is human sexual behaviour fundamentally different from that of other species?
6 Comment on the notion of "female" sex hormones.
7 Consider psychosurgery in the light of inducing a neuropathology to alleviate a behavioural pathology.

Further Readings

Amir, S., Brown, Z.W. and Amit, Z. The role of endorphins in stress: Evidence and speculation. *Neuroscience and Biobehavioral Reviews*, 1980, **4**, 77–86.

Glass, D.C. Stress, behavior patterns and coronary disease. *American Scientist*, 1977, **65**, 177–187.

Goldstein, M. Brain research and violent behavior. *Archives of Neurology*, 1974, **30**, 1–35.

McGeer, P.L. and McGeer, E.C. Chemistry of mood and emotion. *Annual Review of Psychology*, 1980, **31**, 273–307.

Miller, N.E. Learning, stress and psychosomatic symptoms. *Acta Neurobiologica Experimentalis (Warsaw)*, 1976, **36**, 141–156.

Seggie, J. Singhal, R. and Hrdina, P. Animal models and human psychoneuroendocrinology: a selected minireview. *Canadian Journal of Physiology and Pharmacology*, 1980, **58**, 589–599.

Valenstein, E.S. *Brain Control*. New York, Wiley. 1973.

10
Learning and Memory

10.1 Introduction

One of the most useful abilities to have emerged through evolution is the ability to change our behaviour as a result of experience. This process, which is called learning, greatly increases adaptability and allows a broad range of behaviours. Organisms with little or no ability to learn are functionally rigid and have very limited behaviour repertoires. The relative contribution to behaviour of learning as opposed to hereditary factors is a matter of controversy and need not concern us here. In humans, learning is a particularly important determinant of behaviour.

We shall also avoid the thorny issue of defining learning. The definition problems arise in part from attempting to include all those changes in behaviour that obviously involve learning (language acquisition, riding a bicycle, and so on), while excluding more contentious changes such as those that occur during maturation, senility, or following a broken limb.

To demonstrate that learning has taken place, it is necessary to see some change in performance after the learning experience. The persistence of learning over time implicates a storage process, typically called memory. For a memory to be used it must be retrieved from storage. Thus, the demonstration of learning is dependent upon four interrelated factors of which learning is only one. The four factors are learning, storage, retrieval and performance. By the same token, the demonstration of memory is dependent upon the same four factors.

Since these four factors form an interrelated chain, an effect on any link can be confused with an effect on any other. It requires exhaustive experimentation to distinguish between the four factors. In the study of learning and memory, today's spectacular findings are frequently tomorrow's artifacts. However, the potential value of a fundamental understanding of learning and memory is enormous. The steady, if unspectacular progress in this area is a tribute to the ingenuity and persistence of the researchers involved.

10.2 The anatomy of memory

Since learning persists over time as memory, it is reasonable to suppose that memories are stored somewhere. The hypothetical physical representation of a memory is called the *engram* or memory trace. The question that has occupied, or perhaps plagued, memory researchers concerns the location of the engram.

The engram or memory trace is the physical representation of a memory.

Karl Lashley started (and some would say finished) the search for the engram over 50 years ago. His basic paradigm was to teach animals a simple task and then remove various parts of the brain. The rationale behind his approach was that if the engram is removed surgically, the subject will no longer have a memory of the particular learning task. Early research seemed to meet with some success, but the effects were later shown to be artifactual. The apparent loss of memory following various surgical treatments usually reflected a disruption of sensory and motor processes. This interpretive complication should have been expected since the cerebral cortex, which was the area most intensively investigated, had long been known to play a major role in both sensory and motor processes (see Chapter 4). Most research suggests that engrams are distributed widely and, consequently, are remarkably immune to surgical disruption.

Lashley and a generation of subsequent researchers have shown that it is extremely difficult to disrupt a memory surgically.

Apparent surgical disruptions of memory often reflect the non-specific disruptive effects of brain surgery.

Attention has more recently moved away from the cortex to sub-cortical areas. Huston and his colleagues have demonstrated learning in the rat after the removal of the entire neocortex, hippocampus, striatum and amygdala. However, the learning was evident only when simple motor responses, such as head movements or even immobility, were used as responses. If Huston had used more conventional and relatively complex responses such as lever-pressing or maze running, he would have arrived at the erroneous conclusion that learning and the subsequent formation of memories was not possible in the animals.

Rodents, at least, can form memories after total removal of the neocortex, hippocampus, striatum and amygdala.

10.3 The electrophysiology of learning and memory

Since the engram does not appear to be located in a specific, fixed position in the brain, we must examine other storage possibilities. One possibility is that learning activates or opens up new

A difficulty found in all areas of memory research is that of distinguishing physiological or biochemical changes due to learning from the wide variety of changes that can be caused by simple stimulation or activation.

"circuits" in the brain. This switchboard view of memory has been investigated primarily by examining changes in the electrical activity of the brain in order to specify the changes that may have taken place in the switchboard. One problem with this approach is that we do not know what electrophysiological changes to look for, or where to look for them. Nevertheless, electrophysiological investigations have produced some useful findings. For example, there are a number of electrophysiological variables that change in a reasonably predictable manner in response to various environmental changes. The continuing problem is to dissociate learning and memory-induced changes from various non-associative changes in neural activity.

The electroencephalogram or EEG, which is typically recorded from electrodes on the surface of the scalp, is an easily obtained index of brain function. However, the EEG is also an indirect measure which probably reflects a complex mixture of the electrical activity of many millions of neurons and perhaps satellite cells as well. In the resting awake human with eyes closed, the dominant electrical signal is of a high-voltage and rhythmic low-frequency. This fundamental component of the EEG is called alpha-activity. When the eyes are opened suddenly, a striking change occurs. Alpha is replaced by low-voltage, non-rhythmic, high-frequency activity called beta-activity. This electrophysiological change reflects attentional processes, and is called alpha blocking or desynchronization. In so far as attentional processes are necessary to learning, alpha blocking may be seen as an electrophysiological index or correlate of learning. Alpha blocking is also a useful index of arousal (Chapter 6).

Photic driving experiments indicate that the EEG can be classically conditioned.

More direct evidence on electrophysiological involvement in learning and memory processes comes from studies using a technique called photic driving. If a flickering light is presented, the EEG will tend to be "driven" at the same frequency as the flickering light. If the flickering light is then repeatedly paired with another stimulus such as a tone, which, by itself, does not cause EEG driving, eventually the tone, by itself, will cause EEG driving. This is an example of the classical conditioning of an electrophysiological response. The conditioned driving at first appears all over the cortex but eventually becomes restricted to the occipital areas, the areas most clearly implicated in vision.

Memories appear to be simultaneously stored in many different brain sites.

These results could be interpreted as yet another electrophysiological correlate of learning or, more interestingly, they suggest that the EEG learned the new association. There are also recording data from microelectrodes, suggesting that single cells can "learn" to modify their activity. The fact that learning can be demonstrated at all levels, from that of the whole organism to that of single cells, suggests its importance in the integration of behaviour. However, its widespread anatomical distribution makes the phenomenon difficult to investigate. The difficulty is illustrated by research into the role of hippocampal theta in learning and memory processes.

During the early 1960s a number of researchers demonstrated that, during learning tasks, the electrical activity of the hippocampus of cats underwent a regular sequence of changes. The background of fast, low-voltage, desynchronized activity changed to one of slow (5–7 Hz), high-voltage, synchronous activity. The latter rhythm has been found in a number of species and is called the theta-rhythm. There was an immediate flurry of interest in hippocampal theta since damage to the hippocampus in humans produces striking disturbances in memory (see 10.12).

However, in this apparently imminent "marriage" between basic brain research and human neurological findings, hippocampal theta was left standing at the altar. First, theta has been difficult to detect in primates. Second, eliminating theta with drugs appears to have little effect on learning or memory. Perhaps a more serious criticism of the role of theta and the hippocampus in learning is the demonstration of learning and memory in some species after total removal of the hippocampus. More recently, theta has been viewed as an electrophysiological correlate of voluntary movement rather than as an index of learning or memory.

10.4 Electrical disruption of memory processes

Whereas attempts at spatially localizing the engram have been fairly unsuccessful, research into the temporal characteristics of memory formation has been considerably more successful. This research is based on the assumption that the engram does not appear instantaneously as fully developed and mature. Instead, the engram is generally thought to take time to develop, and its fixation may even go through a series of developmental steps corresponding to the formation of short-term and long-term memory. The process of solidifying and elaborating of the engram is referred to as *consolidation*.

Consolidation refers to the development of permanency of an engram.

During consolidation the engram is thought to be vulnerable to disruption, but once consolidation is complete the memory is essentially permanent. During the consolidation process, the engram is commonly thought to exist as a distinct pattern of electrophysiological activity, whereas after consolidation it is probably stored in some biochemical manner. A prediction from this viewpoint is that inhibiting either the relevant electrophysiological or biochemical processes should inhibit memory formation.

While engrams are still consolidating they are thought to be particularly vulnerable to disruption.

The regional abolition of electrophysiological activity (particularly hippocampal theta) is conspicuous for its lack of effect on memory. One reason is that memories are not confined to any one structure, but are represented diffusely at many sites

Electroconvulsive shock (ECS) generates seizure activity which massively disrupts the electrical activity of the brain.

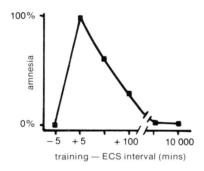

The amnesic effect of electroconvulsive shock (ECS) as a function of the interval between a learning experience and the administration of ECS.

Some of the apparent amnesic effects of ECS may reflect a disruption of memory retrieval processes.

in the brain. This anatomical diffuseness also makes it difficult to record meaningful electrophysiological correlates of learning and memory. In order to record the electrophysiological profile of a memory, it is necessary to know the entire memory "circuit". At present we do not know any complete memory circuits. Moreover, even if we did, they would probably involve so many thousands of neurons that it would be technically impossible to record from more than a small fraction of the relevant cells. The fact that, in the early stages at least, memory is commonly thought to consist of a pattern of electrophysiological changes has important implications. Disruption of electrophysiological activity of the brain should block the formation of memories. However, this blockade should only be effective during the early stages of memory formation.

The most common method for disrupting the electrical activity of the brain is by electroconvulsive shock (ECS). ECS is generally administered by placing electrodes on either side of the head and then passing a short burst of high-frequency and high intensity electrical current through the brain. It should be stressed that ECS is not used experimentally in humans. The human data come from the widespread therapeutic use of ECS in psychiatry (see Chapter 11). Other brain traumas, such as oxygen deprivation, low blood sugar levels or a blow to the head, may also produce a similar net effect. The net effect of all of these brain traumas is a loss of memory (amnesia) for those events occurring just before the trauma. Earlier memories appear to be much less disturbed.

By administering ECS at varying times after a learning task it is possible to plot a temporal gradient of the amnesic effects and, by inference, a gradient of the time taken for the consolidation of a particular memory. Hypothetical results from an idealized ECS experiment are shown in the diagram. Generally, ECS before learning has relatively little effect, indicating that it does not simply disrupt performance. Immediately after learning, ECS produces a strong amnesic effect, but as the learning–ECS interval is lengthened, the effect diminishes rapidly. The shape of the gradient varies markedly as a function of a number of variables, but generally it looks like that in the diagram.

Whereas the amnesic effect of ECS is most commonly attributed to a disruption of memory, some findings suggest an interference with retrieval processes. The latter interpretation arises from the apparent lack of permanency of ECS-induced amnesia in some circumstances. If ECS simply blocks consolidation, then the memory should never reach storage. However, in certain cases the memory seems to recover spontaneously over time, or it can be reinstated by a "reminder" cue. The impermanence of amnesia and the ability to reinstate memory with reminding cues suggest that ECS may not always prevent memory storage. The apparent disruption of memory produced by ECS under some circumstances may instead represent an interference with retrieval processes. This may be analogous with having something "on the tip of one's tongue" but not being able to say it. However, in many cases ECS-induced amnesia is permanent and no amount of "reminding" will reinstate the memory.

Several recent experiments with ECS have suggested that the development of tolerance to narcotics may be a form of learning. Tolerance refers to the diminished effectiveness of a given drug dose when given repeatedly. For example, the analgesic or pain-reducing effect of morphine is lessened by just one previous exposure to the drug. However, if the previous administration is followed immediately by ECS, no tolerance develops. It is as if the ECS causes the animal to "forget" the previous exposure. If the ECS is given before, or well after, the initial morphine exposure it has no effect on the development of tolerance.

Drug tolerance may be mediated by cellular level memory since ECS may block the formation of drug tolerance.

10.5 The biochemistry of learning and memory

It is generally accepted that long-term memories are preserved as some relatively stable biochemical change. Whatever the nature of the storage process, it probably involves altered functional connections among neurons. For this reason most research into the biochemical basis of memory has been concerned with the constituents of the cell membrane (proteins), or of the cell's metabolic apparatus (nucleic acids), or with neurotransmitters themselves (peptides). These chemicals by no means exhaust the possibilities for long-term modulation of neurotransmission. They are merely the currently favoured substances.

It is widely thought that long-term memories are stored as some biochemical change.

The involvement of biochemicals in memory has been investigated in a number of ways including (1) the study of biochemical and structural changes in the brain, (2) altering memory by the use of drugs and (3) transfer of memory by cannibalism and brain extracts. When different methods are used in conjunction with the multiplicity of learning tasks available, and a wide range of species are studied, it is not surprising that the literature contains many contradictory, unreplicated and improbable findings. Both structurally and biochemically, the brain is changed by experience. However, unequivocally associating these changes with learning and memory has been more difficult.

10.6 Is the brain modified by experience?

An optimistic approach to the extreme individual differences in learning ability is that they reflect the influences of different environments. A more pessimistic approach is to attribute the differences in learning ability to genetic factors. This latter view

Although the brain is modified by experience, it has been extremely difficult to ascertain which modifications are due to learning as opposed to stimulation and activation.

Environmental deprivation in rats produces anatomical, biochemical and functional changes in the brain.

is pessimistic since, once something is interpreted as being due to genetic factors, there is little impetus to further research, or to attempts to modify that characteristic.

Perhaps the first evidence showing that the brain is modified by experience was provided in a series of experiments by Bennett, Diamond, Krech and Rosenzweig. They were interested in the relative effects on brain structure and biochemistry of rearing rats in either an enriched or impoverished environment. The potential social importance of their research should be obvious. At the gross anatomical level, they found that the enrichment condition increased the thickness and weight of the cerebral cortex. At the microanatomical level, the size of the cortical neurons increased, as did the size and perhaps number of synaptic contacts with other neurons. At the biochemical level, they found that enrichment increased the quantity of acetylcholinesterase, the enzyme responsible for the breakdown of the neurotransmitter acetylcholine.

Overall, the rats that experienced early environmental enrichment were anatomically and biochemically superior to, or at least different from, those in the deprived group. Perhaps the most socially provocative aspect of their research is the finding that the adverse effects of a poor early environment could be reversed. In adolescence or early adulthood, exposure to the enriched environment could reverse the anatomical and biochemical deficiencies resulting from an environmentally-impoverished childhood. Unfortunately, relating the brain changes to behaviour, particularly learning, has not been straightforward.

10.7 Biochemistry made easy

It is thought that long-term memories are preserved as unique biochemical entities for two reasons. First, electrophysiological activity is generally seen as having insufficient long-term stability to serve as a permanent storage mechanism. Second, because biochemical substances such as proteins are complex aggregations of some 20 different constituent amino acids, their variety is practically infinite. In other words, they have the potential to 'code' every single experience as a unique molecule.

However, neither assumption supporting an exclusive emphasis on biochemical rather than electrophysiological coding of long-term memory is well founded. Nothing is known about the relative fragility of electrophysiological, compared with biochemical, activity. In addition, since there are at least 10^{10} neurons in the brain, each of which can, in the simplest case, be either active or non-active, the total number of possible different brain states is 10^{10^9}, a number much greater than the total number of particles in the universe. Consequently, the coding potential of our electrophysiological switchboard is essentially infinite. However, since there is virtually no information on electrophysiological mechanisms of long-term memory, we shall restrict our discussion to biochemical mechanisms.

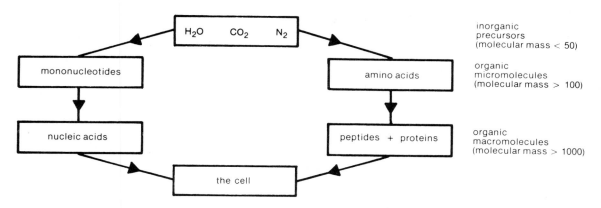

Simplified illustration of some general relations among the basic elements (water, carbon dioxide and nitrogen), micromolecules, macromolecules and a living structure, the cell.

In order to appreciate the elegance and difficulties of the biochemical line of research, we need to know a few biochemical terms. We shall concentrate on the general relationship between amino acids, nucleic acids, proteins and peptides.

An examination of the molecular masses at the various stages of the diagram indicates that the first substantial information-coding potential is found at the level of the organic macromolecules. This ability is illustrated well by deoxyribonucleic acid (DNA) which contains the genetic code. However, because of its relative stability, it is unlikely that DNA codes the rapidly changing environmental information required for memory. For this reason, attention has centred on ribonucleic acid (RNA), peptides and proteins. In the simplest sense the relationship between the macromolecules is as follows. DNA directs the synthesis of RNA from nucleotides, and RNA directs the synthesis of proteins from amino acids. Peptides may be seen as sub-units of proteins, since they are smaller and less complex combinations of amino acids.

There are two apparently direct ways to investigate the possibility that organic macromolecules are involved in memory. First, learning should result in changes in the macromolecules in the brain. Second, interfering with macromolecule synthesis should impair memory. Some support is indicated for both predictions. However it is difficult to associate these effects unequivocally with memory processes, rather than with non-associative changes produced by environmental stimulation and arousal.

10.8 Changes in RNA and proteins following learning

The first systematic examination of the quantitative and qualitative changes in RNA during learning was conducted by Hydén and colleagues in Sweden. In rats that had learned to climb an elevated wire, RNA was altered in some of the vestibular system neurons. The control group was given passive vestibular stimulation by being placed in an automated swing. Difficulty in interpreting the results arises from the fact that the two types of vestibular stimulation (balancing and swinging) are obviously different. Consequently, the biochemical differences between the experimental and control groups might simply reflect different types of sensory stimulation and not differences in learning.

Hydén also reported an increase in the brain-specific protein S-100 in rats trained to use their non-preferred paw (rats are right- or left-pawed). More impressively, the anti-serum to S-100 prevented further learning of the task without producing a general motor impairment. However, the findings could reflect the use of new components of the motor system and not an effect on learning or memory. While there have been many other experiments along similar lines, they are all at least partly subject to similar methodological criticisms.

10.9 Inhibition of RNA synthesis

RNA synthesis inhibitors often produce toxic side effects which may be confused with a disruption in memory.

Among the drugs effective in blocking the synthesis of RNA are the antibiotics actinomycin-D and 8-azaguanine. Such a basic disruption of biological processes should have widespread physiological repercussions. This is usually the case. These and other antibiotics are toxic compounds, and even when they are used therapeutically the physician is trading-off a therapeutic effect against a host of undesirable side effects.

The problem is that since the doses of antibiotics required to substantially inhibit RNA synthesis are high, they usually make the experimental subject sick. Consequently, any apparent loss in memory could be due either to the inhibition of RNA synthesis or to making the subject sick. In spite of undesirable side effects, a number of researchers have reported that inhibition of RNA synthesis has no effect on either learning or memory. Because of these and other difficulties with investigating memory coding by RNA, many investigators have turned to the study of proteins.

10.10 Inhibition of protein synthesis

If the consolidation of the engram involves the formation of memory-specific proteins, then disrupting the process should impair memory. The logic here is essentially the same as that employed in the case of other amnesic treatments such as ECS or inhibition of RNA synthesis. The use of synthesis-inhibitors such as puromycin provided early support for this view. However, as for several other aspects of the biochemistry of memory, later research has suggested a different interpretation.

In several species direct intracerebral injection of puromycin results in amnesia. The effect is produced when the injections are given up to 2 days after the learning task. However, even if puromycin could be shown to have no effect on motor performance as such, the results are still subject to interpretational difficulties. First, as was the case with ECS, the amnesia produced by puromycin is not always permanent. In some cases an intracerebral injection of water can apparently restore the memory. More important, other more potent protein-synthesis inhibitors may actually block the amnesic effect of puromycin.

Intracerebral injections of the protein synthesis inhibitor puromycin produce amnesia much like that produced by ECS. They both may work by disrupting the electrical activity of the brain.

These results indicate that the amnesic effect of puromycin is not due simply to inhibiting protein synthesis, so the question of why puromycin produces amnesia remains. Since the effect of puromycin on memory may be reversible, it would probably be more appropriate to rephrase the question. How does puromycin disrupt the retrieval of memory? The principal difference between the effect of puromycin and the other protein-synthesis inhibitors that are less effective in producing amnesia is that puromycin, like ECS, produces a profound disruption of the electrical activity of the brain. It is possible that the electrophysiological disruption, and not the inhibition of protein synthesis is responsible for the apparent amnesia produced by puromycin.

More direct results implicating protein synthesis in memory, or at least retrieval processes, come from experiments using the protein-synthesis inhibitor anisomycin. The anisomycin data are somewhat easier to interpret than those of other synthesis inhibitors because anisomycin produces relatively mild side effects. There are also recent data indicating that drugs which interfere with the uptake of amino acids into cells may selectively interfere with either memory retrieval or formation.

10.11 Transfer of memory

If memories are coded by some change in macromolecular configuration, and if we could isolate the macromolecules and administer them to the relevant sites in another organism, and if that subject could "decode" the macromolecules, then we may be able to "transfer" a memory from one subject to another. Given this host of largely unsupported assumptions the issue of memory-transfer remains the wild and woolly frontier of

The transfer of memory by organic macromolecules remains the most disputed area of memory research.

memory research. However, such theoretical objections do not constitute an adequate reason for rejecting this research approach out of hand. If transfer of memory can be demonstrated unequivocally, then our current lack of knowledge concerning the possible mechanisms of transfer becomes simply another intellectual problem.

Another largely invalid criticism of memory-transfer research is based on the distressingly frequent failure to replicate some of the basic experimental findings. The failures are sometimes used to obscure the fact that all of the basic findings have been replicated at least occasionally, and by reputable investigators. Emerging from this research is a growing number of findings suggesting that it is possible to transfer at least something via brain extracts. Whether this something is memory or an entirely different capacity remains unclear.

There are two main techniques for investigating memory transfer. One involves cannibalism, which commonly occurs in some species of flatworms. The other involves the extraction of various macromolecules from the brain of a trained subject and their injection into an untrained subject. In either case a transfer effect is shown if the ingestion or injection facilitates the learning of the task in a naive subject. However, the effect must be measured in relation to that shown by appropriate control subjects.

A persistent problem in memory research is the use of appropriate control groups.

Early research was characterized by a lack of controls, appropriate or otherwise. Recent research has recognized this inadequacy, but it is still plagued by the problem of what constitutes an appropriate control. For example, let us assume that a brain extract from a rat trained in shock avoidance was shown to facilitate shock-avoidance learning in a naive rat. Unless extracts from untrained rats were also used, the facilitation might reflect simply a stimulant effect of the brain extract. However, even if the facilitation were shown to be greater than that produced by the extract from a rat not trained in shock avoidance, the difference might reflect the fact that the electric shock has increased the stimulant value of the brain extract.

Perhaps an appropriate control "donor" would be a rat that had received a similar number of similarly spaced shocks. Yet even this is not adequate, since any different effect might reflect the fact that one rat was active and could control the shock, whereas the other was shocked in a behaviour-independent manner. An ideal control would be a subject that received the same amount of stimulation, while behaving in the same way yet did not learn anything. Of course, this is impossible since some learning probably takes place in any situation. However, even if all that can be transferred is sensitization, activation or a vague behavioural tendency, it still remains an interesting phenomenon.

10.12 Human memory disorders

The human brain is bilaterally symmetrical. This is particularly obvious at the level of the cerebral cortex (see Chapter 4). Anatomical symmetry is contrasted with a clear-cut functional asymmetry, again particularly at the level of the cerebral cortex. In most humans, the left hemisphere is most important for language functions, whereas the right hemisphere is "dominant" for spatial abilities. It is not surprising then that cortical damage on one side can produce a variety of functional deficits. What is surprising is that, in sharp contrast to the non-specific memory deficits seen in laboratory species, many human memory deficits produced by cortical damage are remarkably specific.

The memory deficits produced by brain damage in humans are usually far more specific than those seen in laboratory animals.

The classic case in the literature is a person known only as H.M. In order to alleviate an incapacitating case of epilepsy, surgeons carried out bilateral temporal lobe lesions on H.M. The principal structure destroyed was the hippocampus. Following the operation, H.M. showed a complete and permanent inability to acquire long-term memory. Both his preoperative memories and his ability to form short-term memories were largely unaffected.

Destruction of the human hippocampus results in the loss of ability to form permanent memories.

Similarly, his overall intelligence seemed unimpaired. For example, he could retain a three digit number only by continuously repeating a complex and intellectually demanding mnemonic. As soon as he stopped the repetition, he not only forgot the number, but he was totally unaware that he had been asked to remember anything. He could remember his former presurgical address, but he had no idea of his new post-surgical one. Nor did he remember that he and his family had moved. His deficit was most poignantly described by himself ". . . at this moment everything looks clear to me, but what happened before? That's what worries me. It's like waking from a dream. I just don't remember."

A further peculiarity of the memory disorder shown by H.M. suggested that verbal and motor memories involve different brain mechanisms. For example, on a mirror-image drawing task H.M. showed a progressive improvement over repeated daily sessions, even though he could not remember ever having done the task before. That is, his perceptual–motor memory of the task was unimpaired even though he had no verbal memory at all.

Verbal and motor memories can be independently affected by certain types of brain damage.

Further specialization of memory processes is suggested by results from patients with damage restricted to the left temporal lobe. When a sequence of letters was presented verbally to one patient, he showed virtually no memory of the sequence. However, when the same sequence was presented visually, his memory was essentially unimpaired. There are also cases showing a converse deficit: some people can remember material presented verbally but not material presented visually.

Thus we see that the language abilities of humans add a further dimension of complexity to the issue of the physiological basis of memory. It seems that language and spatial–musical abilities are served by different mechanisms. Even within the area of language memory, there appear to be fundamental distinctions between long-term and short-term memory. Similarly, there may be quite different mechanisms involved in the memory of material presented in the visual as opposed to the auditory manner.

Questions

1   Consider the logic of having a "memory centre" in the brain.
2   Why should the surface EEG have little to tell us about learning or memory?
3   Discuss the problems of determining the existence of a memory molecule.
4   Design an experiment to distinguish between a true amnesiac effect and a disruption of memory retrieval.
5   Why should there be separate processes for short-term and long-term memory?
6   How can physiological trauma produce loss of memory in humans?
7   Totally amnesic humans do not forget how to walk or talk. What does this indicate about the nature of memory storage?

Further Readings

Barraco, R.A. and Stettner, L.J. Antibiotics and memory. *Psychological Bulletin*, 1976, **83**, 242–302.
Dunn, A.J. Neurochemistry of learning and memory: An evaluation of recent data. *Annual Review of Psychology*, 1980, **31**, 343–390.
Horn, G., Rose, S.P.R. and Bateson, P.P.G. Experience and plasticity in the central nervous system. *Science*, 1973, **181**, 506–514.
Riley, A.L., Zelker, D.A. and Duncan, H.J. The role of endorphins in animal learning and behavior. *Neuroscience and Biobehavioral Reviews*, 1980, **4**, 69–76.
Thompson, R.F. The search for the engram. *American Psychologist*, 1976, **31**, 209–227.

11

The Biological Basis of Psychiatry

11.1 Introduction

In most cases when people seek or need psychiatric assistance, the psychiatric disability is relatively mild and transient. In other cases the disability, while transient, is great enough to prevent the patient fulfilling his normal functions. There remain many people who are condemned to a life of almost complete dysfunction. They populate the fringes of our society and the wards of our psychiatric institutions. They are grim reminders of the extent to which living can be dehumanized. It is not surprising that some choose self-destruction, or engage in violence upon others. Apart from this, the psychiatrically impaired constitute an ocean of misery, the understanding of which must be among our highest social priorities.

Before describing the contributions made to psychiatry by the neurosciences, we shall point to areas where this approach has little to contribute. Just as pills and potions cure many physiological maladies, it may appear reasonable that a similar approach should be successful with behavioural problems. However, many behavioural problems are due to deficient or wrongly directed learning and can only be cured by re-learning. No pill can replace learning, but the ease of "popping a pill" often appeals when compared to slower methods of behaviour change.

On the other hand, physiological treatments are clearly appropriate for some psychiatric problems. With these treatments, true "cures" are, as yet, rare. Usually, there is only temporary or partial remission of symptoms. With the two major psychoses, schizophrenia and manic-depression, traditional psychotherapy has been largely ineffective. Improvements due to behaviour

Although many psychiatric problems do not represent a physiological pathology, the major psychoses have a prominent physiological component.

modification techniques, while significant, often do little more than make patients better custodial cases. The primary symptoms of the psychoses remain largely unaffected. These and other considerations suggest that the major psychoses have a primary biological basis.

SCHIZOPHRENIA

11.2 Description

Schizophrenia is the major cause for psychiatric institutionalization throughout the world. As with many other psychiatric diagnostic categories, the definition and diagnosis of schizophrenia is imprecise. Thus there is considerable controversy about the main features of the disease.

Schizophrenia has nothing to do with the split-personality depicted in movies.

An emerging view is that schizophrenia may not be a single disease. The trend is to speak of the "group of schizophrenias" as did Bleuler, who coined the term originally. Schizophrenia may thus represent a number of diverse disorders with different aetiologies and different appropriate treatments. A similar transition has been made with the general medical concept of anaemia. While it began as a unitary concept, anaemia has not become differentiated into distinct subtypes with regard to aetiology, symptomatology and treatment.

In contrast to anaemia, the differentiation of schizophrenic subtypes is more controversial. From as few as two to as many as nine different subtypes have been differentiated by various investigators. Furthermore, the relevant characteristics of schizophrenia are not agreed upon. Some clinicians stress the importance of speed of onset of the disease or the presence of delusional patterns, whereas others may stress the amount of motor activity displayed by the patient. The different points of emphasis have suggested the following dimensions of schizophrenia: acute-chronic, paranoid-non-paranoid, and agitated-stuporous. They are not the only relevant dimensions, but they exemplify the complexity of the problem. For simplicity we consider the following as the core symptoms of the schizophrenias: (1) blunting of affect; (2) withdrawal from reality; and (3) thought disorders.

Schizophrenia is a poorly defined group of dysfunctions the symptoms of which include: (1) blunting of affect; (2) withdrawal from reality; and (3) thought disorders.

Symptoms such as hallucinations and paranoia lend themselves better to dramatic representation. In movies, asylums are often populated by Napoleons and Jesi, or by quaint people who converse with non-existent companions. However, such symptoms are generally considered to be less important because they do not impair everyday functioning as much as the core symptoms do.

Although auditory hallucinations are one of the more florid symptoms of schizophrenia, many clinicians feel they are secondary, not primary, components of the disease.

We shall now consider evidence suggesting that the schizophrenias have a primary biological basis.

11.3 Genetic factors in schizophrenia

There is evidence to suggest a strong genetic contribution to schizophrenia; that is, schizophrenia tends to "run in families". It has been argued that a high incidence of schizophrenia in a family may merely indicate that people raised in a disturbed environment tend to become disturbed. However, this alone cannot explain the genetic contribution. For example, one study found that in 11 pairs of monozygotic (identical) twins separated before their first birthday, 8 pairs were fully concordant (both twins were schizophrenic), whereas 2 of the 3 remaining pairs were partially concordant (that is, one twin was schizophrenic and the other "borderline" schizophrenic).

Overall, the combined results of many studies suggest that dizygotic (non-identical) twins show a concordance rate for schizophrenia of about 10%, whereas in monozygotic twins the rate is well over 40%. The latter figure is greater than the concordance rate in monozygotic twins for diabetes, which is unquestionably a physiological pathology.

There is a strong genetic component to schizophrenia.

11.4 Is schizophrenia due to a biochemical abnormality?

Perhaps the most persuasive evidence for a biological basis of schizophrenia comes from demonstrations that certain drugs can either induce schizophrenia-like states or alleviate the symptoms of naturally occurring schizophrenia. These findings provide strong, but still indirect, evidence that schizophrenia is caused by an underlying biochemical abnormality. Direct evidence for a biochemical abnormality can only be provided by analysing tissue and bodily fluids of schizophrenics. We will see below that, whereas the indirect evidence for a biochemical abnormality is overwhelming (11.8), the direct evidence is less conclusive (11.6).

11.5 Biochemically inducing schizophrenia

A variety of naturally occurring diseases and poisons may produce psychiatric symptoms somewhat similar to those of schizophrenia. However, people suffering from these diseases or toxic states are typically in a state of general delirium and often do not know where they are, or what time it is. In contrast, a schizophrenic is typically relatively well oriented with respect to space and time. The delirious person has a vague or non-existent sense of reality, whereas the schizophrenic often has an acute, but terribly twisted sense of reality.

A classic case of diagnostic confusion occurred in the southern

The vitamin B deficiency disease pellagra was once widely confused with schizophrenia.

Hallucinogenic and 'recreational' drugs such as LSD and cannabis have been erroneously labelled as psychotomimetic. The states they produce bear little resemblance to naturally occurring psychoses.

Strong stimulant drugs such as amphetamine can produce a state that closely resembles the paranoid form of schizophrenia.

The abuse of stimulant drugs is strongly associated with crimes of violence.

United States with the vitamin B deficiency disease *pellagra*. At one time, as many as 10% of the population in southern mental hospitals were diagnosed as schizophrenic when they were actually suffering from pellagra. Massive vitamin B treatments quickly cured pellagra, and there was hope that a similarly effective cure would be found for schizophrenia. Enriching bread with vitamin B has virtually eradicated pellagra, but schizophrenia has turned out to be a far more difficult problem.

There are other pharmacologically induced states which bear a closer resemblance to schizophrenia. For example, the mesquite cactus, peyote buds, indian hemp and lysergic acid can induce hallucinations and other perceptual–emotional changes. The states produced by these substances have been said to be "model" psychoses, and the substances were once widely referred to as *psychotomimetic*. However, it now appears that the altered states of consciousness produced by these drugs are different from the psychotic dysfunction of schizophrenia. This has been demonstrated by administering lysergic acid diethylamide (LSD) to schizophrenics.

If LSD were psychotomimetic, it would be expected to exaggerate schizophrenic symptoms. However, all the drug did was to produce a "tripping" schizophrenic. These individuals could differentiate the drug-induced state from their ongoing psychosis. Further, hallucinogenic drugs generally produce visual hallucinations, whereas the hallucinations of schizophrenics are almost always auditory — they hear "voices". Such considerations suggest that the effects of hallucinogenic drugs probably have little relevance to schizophrenia.

In contrast with the hallucinogens, the effects of some stimulant-euphoriant drugs are very relevant to schizophrenia. The continuous use of even moderate doses of amphetamine or cocaine over some days can produce a state clinically indistinguishable from paranoid schizophrenia. These people ("speed-freaks") become suspicious and withdrawn, convinced that they are the target of some evil and insidious conspiracy, they hear voices that tell them to do strange, sometimes violent things, and they frequently develop hallucinations, both auditory and tactile. The drug-induced paranoid state may result in elaborate schemes of self-protection.

One amphetamine enthusiast was found wearing rubber gloves, a rubber face-mask and goggles. He carried several knives, pistols and a hand grenade. Underneath his clothes he wore a complete rubber wet-suit. He said the rubber clothing was necessary since he knew that "they" were after him, and when they caught up with him, they were planning to throw acid on him. Amphetamine and cocaine users are often involved in crimes of violence, which they view as being purely defensive — "If I don't get them first, they'll get me."

Amphetamine-psychosis is not only found in chronic drug users. It has been demonstrated in psychiatrically normal volunteers with no history of drug abuse. If amphetamine is administered to hospitalized schizophrenics, it produces an immediate worsening of schizophrenic symptoms. In schizophrenics who are in remission, that is who currently have no symptoms, amphetamine can provoke a rapid return to schizophrenic behaviour.

Amphetamine can only produce the paranoid form of schizophrenia, which suggests that there are biochemically different subgroups of schizophrenia. If we can determine the effect amphetamine has on the brain, we may be able to counteract its effects and, by inference, counteract naturally occurring schizophrenias. This approach has been partly successful. However, even if the neurochemical changes brought about by an amphetamine or therapeutic drug were completely specified, there remains a major conceptual problem. For example, we will see below that anti-schizophrenic drugs generally reduce dopaminergic activity in the brain. The inference commonly drawn from this is that schizophrenia is caused by excessive dopaminergic activity. This seemingly straightforward logic has an important flaw which can be illustrated by the following example. If you were somewhat nervous before a social engagement, a few drinks would likely have a positive therapeutic effect. It would not, however, be reasonable to conclude that the cause of your nervousness was an inadequate level of alcohol in the brain. In other words, an effective therapy does not necessarily indicate the aetiology of the disease.

11.6 Biochemical abnormalities in schizophrenics

As mentioned in 11.4, direct evidence for a biochemical basis of schizophrenia requires the demonstration of some biochemical abnormality in schizophrenics. There have been a number of approaches to this problem, all of which have generated rather equivocal results.

The most direct attack on this problem is to biochemically assay the brains of schizophrenics. Besides the obvious difficulty of requiring the researcher to wait for the death of sufficient numbers of schizophrenics, this approach has other severe limitations. Patients vary widely in terms of age, severity of schizophrenia, general health, medication and diet. In addition, widely varying times between death and the biochemical analysis, as well as the varying sensitivities of different analytic techniques make such data subject to many potential artifacts. The confused and conflicting reports in this area well reflect the above methodological difficulties.

Clinically usable measures of the biochemical activity of the brain are very indirect and consequently imprecise.

The functional state of a given neurotransmitter system is determined jointly by transmitter availability and receptor sensitivity.

The biochemical state of the brain can also be indirectly measured in living patients by analysing blood, urine and cerebrospinal fluid. The logic behind this approach is that abnormal neurotransmitter activity will be reflected in abnormal levels of neurotransmitters, their enzymes or metabolites in the fluids which serve the brain. Since these fluid-analytic techniques are relatively easily applied they have generated large amounts of data. Unfortunately, the findings are too rarely replicated and too frequently contradicted. The fluid-analytic approach has yet to specify the biochemical abnormality that underlies schizophrenia.

A recurring conceptual problem is the "too much or too little" logic. There is a widespread belief that the functional state of a particular neurotransmitter system will be reflected in the levels of the neurotransmitters, their enzymes or metabolites. In other words, abnormal functional activity must be due to too much or too little of these substances. However, there is an increasing body of evidence which suggests the levels of these substances frequently do not provide an accurate index of the functional state of the system. There can be large changes in levels without any change in the activity of the system. Conversely, there can be large changes in activity without any change in levels of the neurotransmitters, their enzymes or metabolites.

The fact that the activity of a neurotransmitter system does not necessarily reflect the levels of neurotransmitters, their enzymes or metabolites suggests that there must be another means of modulating activity. This additional modulating factor is the excitability and number of neurotransmitter receptors. Changes in receptor number and excitability can produce large changes in activity quite independently of any changes in transmitter availability. Increased receptor numbers or sensitivity can increase functional activity, whereas decreased receptor numbers or sensitivity can decrease activity.

Neurotransmitter receptor changes offer the exciting promise of providing an explanation for the typically slow onset of the therapeutic effects of anti-schizophrenic drugs. The therapeutic effect of most anti-schizophrenic drugs occurs days, weeks or even months after they produce large changes in transmitter availability. On the other hand, these drugs may also produce changes in receptor numbers or excitability which have a slow onset that more closely coincides with the onset of their therapeutic effect. In this vein is the recent report that schizophrenics who had been drug-free for at least a year before their death showed increased density of dopamine receptors in the brain. This could well produce dopaminergic hyperactivity in the presence of normal or even subnormal dopamine levels (see 11.8, 11.9, 11.10).

There is still another recent line of evidence which is also suggestive of an underlying biochemical abnormality as the cause of schizophrenia. If there is a blood-borne factor which exerts a schizophrenic influence on the brain, it may be possible to isolate it and remove it from the schizophrenic's blood. Attempts at identifying such a factor have met with little success, but there are now a few reports of encouraging results with blood filtering. Purifying the blood by dialysis has been reported to have a therapeutic effect in a number of schizophrenics who had not responded satisfactorily to drug therapy. None of these studies were methodologically adequate since they did not control for placebo effects and the experimenters evaluated the patients themselves (see 9.21). Even so, these are provocative findings which will certainly be pursued.

11.7 Managing schizophrenia with drugs

The best information implicating a biochemical defect in schizophrenia stems from the pharmacological management of the disease. The discovery of drugs that substantially alleviate schizophrenic symptoms is one of the great discoveries of this century. Millions of people, formerly condemned to institutions, are now functioning in a relatively "normal" manner. The drugs still do not cure schizophrenia as vitamin B cured pellagra. They do, however, reduce symptoms to such an extent that many patients can resume useful and rewarding lives.

Anti-schizophrenic drugs are collectively referred to as neuroleptics.

Major classes of anti-schizophrenic (neuroleptic) drugs.

	GENERIC NAME	TRADE NAME
Phenothiazines	chlorpromazine thioridazine fluphenazine	Thorazine Mellaril Prolixin
Butyrophenones	haloperidol methylperidol	Haldol Luvatrin
Thioxanthenes	chlorprothixene thiothixene	Taractan Navane
Miscellaneous or atypical	clozapine butaclamol	Leponex

Further, anti-schizophrenic drugs are not simply pharmacological bludgeons that render schizophrenics incapable of displaying any symptoms. Strong sedatives and tranquilizers produce a sedated schizophrenic in whom the blunting of affect, withdrawl and thought disorders continue unabated. Consequently, although anti-schizophrenic drugs were once widely referred to as *major tranquilizers* the term is misleading and is no longer appropriate. Anti-schizophrenic agents are now referred to as *neuroleptics*.

While neuroleptics differ in their mode of neurochemical action, they share the common ability to reduce the activity of dopamine (DA) in the brain. Schizophrenia may thus be due primarily to overactivity in DA neurotransmission. Supporting this hypothesis are studies which show that agents such as amphetamine, which increase DA activity, act to exacerbate or even induce schizophrenia (see 11.5). Further, neuroleptics such as chlorpromazine can prevent the occurrence of, or reverse, amphetamine psychosis.

11.8 Schizophrenia and Parkinson's disease — mirror image disorders?

If schizophrenia is a DA-overactivity disease, it should be interesting to compare it with Parkinson's disease, which appears to be a DA-underactivity disease. The principal symptoms of Parkinson's disease are: (1) akinesia, a difficulty in initiating movements; (2) postural rigidity; and (3) resting tremor. In postmortem histological material from Parkinsonian patients, there is a degeneration of a particular group of DA-containing neurons in the brain.

The cell bodies of the main group of DA neurons relevant to Parkinson's disease originate in an area of the ventral tegmentum called the *substantia nigra*. The axons of the neurons project anteriorly through the hypothalamus, and terminate in the *corpus striatum*. This system is called the *nigro-striatal DA system*, and Parkinson's disease is sometimes called a nigro-striatal DA-deficiency syndrome. The nigro-striatal DA system is a major component of the extra-pyramidal motor system, and Parkinson's disease is one of a larger group of extra-pyramidal motor disorders.

We can make some predictions from the assumption that schizophrenia and Parkinson's disease are mirror-image diseases. First, Parkinson's disease should be exacerbated by anti-schizophrenic drugs, whereas schizophrenia should be exacerbated by anti-Parkinsonian drugs. In general this is true, since neuroleptics exacerbate Parkinson's disease, whereas L-DOPA, the most widely used treatment for Parkinson's disease, may exacerbate schizophrenia.

The ability of typical neuroleptics to induce Parkinsonian-like extra-pyramidal motor dysfunctions, is an undesirable side-effect. To a certain extent, the physician is exchanging schizo-

Schizophrenia has been characterized as a DA overactivity disease, whereas Parkinson's disease is widely thought to involve DA underactivity.

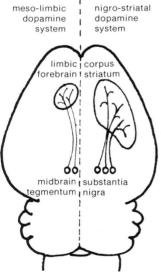

Illustration of the two ascending dopamine systems which have been implicated in schizophrenia (meso-limbic) and Parkinson's disease (nigro-striatal). The illustration is of the rat brain and the view is looking down from the top of the skull. For simplicity each system is only shown on one side of the brain.

phrenia for Parkinson's disease. For a long time many physicians increased neuroleptic dosage progressively until extra-pyramidal side-effects occurred, since it was thought they indicated the effective dose levels for the anti-schizophrenic activity. This practice was based on the notion that schizophrenia and Parkinson's disease represent opposite poles of nigro-striatal DA dysfunction. Recent results indicate that this view is no longer tenable and that the two diseases probably involve different neurochemical systems. Further, the nature of schizophrenia is more complex than a simple DA-overactivity syndrome.

Typical neuroleptics block dopamine receptors and consequently produce Parkinsonian-like motor disturbances.

Whereas the Parkinsonian-like side effects of neuroleptic drugs appear quite rapidly, there is another and more serious group of motor disorders that may only appear after months or even years of drug treatment. These late-appearing motor disorders are called *tardive dyskinesias*. Typically, they take the form of slow twisting movements or rapid twitches of the mouth, tongue, face and head. In contrast to the Parkinsonian-like side effects of neuroleptics, the tardive dyskinesias appear to be largely irreversible. Their irreversibility suggests that long-term neuroleptic medication probably produces permanent changes in brain dopamine receptors.

Long-term neuroleptic use sometimes produces non-Parkinsonian motor disturbances called tardive dyskinesias.

11.9 Which dopamine system?

The first indication that schizophrenia may not simply be a nigro-striatal overactivity syndrome comes from the therapeutic effects of some atypical neuroleptics. For example, *clozapine* has all the anti-schizophrenic ability of the traditional neuroleptics, but produces no extra-pyramidal side effects. Further, there are clinical reports of schizophrenia and Parkinson's disease co-existing in the same patient.

Since most indicators point to some sort of DA disorder in schizophrenia, recent attention has shifted to another group of DA neurons in the brain — the *meso-limbic DA system*. The cell bodies of the meso-limbic DA system originate in the mesencephalon, medial to the substantia nigra. Their axons project anteriorly through the hypothalamus, where they terminate diffusely in several limbic forebrain and frontal cortical areas.

The meso-limbic DA system appears to be more involved in schizophrenia, whereas the nigro-striatal DA system is more involved with motor dysfunctions.

Studies with laboratory animals indicate that typical and atypical neuroleptics differ markedly in their ability to block DA receptors in the two DA systems. Both classes of neuroleptics have approximately equal ability to block meso-limbic DA receptors, whereas only the typical neuroleptics block the nigro-striatal DA receptors substantially. These results led to the suggestion that schizophrenia represents a disorder in the meso-limbic DA system. Since typical neuroleptics block receptors in both DA systems rather indiscriminately, they inevitably

Typical neuroleptics usually antagonize both DA systems, whereas atypical neuroleptics such as clozapine produce a relatively specific antagonism of the meso-limbic DA system.

produce extra-pyramidal side effects. When DA receptor blockade is largely restricted to the meso-limbic system, an anti-schizophrenic effect is achieved without the occurrence of extra-pyramidal motor dysfunction. This is the case with neuroleptics such as clozapine and thioridazine.

11.10 Evidence against the dopamine-overactivity hypothesis of schizophrenia

The amphetamine psychosis and the anti-schizophrenic effect of DA receptor blockers are interpreted as supporting the hypothesis that schizophrenia is due to overactivity in the meso-limbic DA system. However, recent evidence has questioned the validity of this hypothesis.

Analysis of CSF suggests that the DA systems of schizophrenics may be underactive. This is the opposite of what the commonly accepted DA overactivity hypothesis would predict.

Analysis of body fluids of schizophrenics has provided little evidence of DA overactivity (11.6). Recent analyses of the cerebrospinal fluid of schizophrenics indicate that the DA systems in these individuals may actually be underactive. This is the reverse of the DA-overactivity hypothesis. Further, inducing overactivity in DA neurons by the DA receptor stimulant *apomorphine* does not induce any psychotic symptoms. Finally, there have been suggestions that meso-limbic DA receptors may be blocked by a number of drugs that have no anti-schizophrenic effect. However, such discordant findings often give rise to new directions in future research. They raise the prospect that the next few years will see major breakthroughs in this important area.

AFFECTIVE DISORDERS

11.11 Description

The two main components of the affective disorders are depression and mania.

After the schizophrenias, the most common cause for psychiatric institutionalization is a group of disturbances called *affective disorders*. This group includes a variety of disorders representing varying degrees and combinations of *depression* and *mania*. Typical depressive symptoms are lowering of mood, feelings of guilt and hopelessness, and reduced activity and reactivity. Typical manic symptoms are elevation of mood, talkativeness and grandiosity, and enhanced activity and reactivity. Although any of the symptoms can occur during normal mood-swings, it is their magnitude and recurring nature that indicates a psychiatric problem. A severely depressed individual becomes nonfunctional and may attempt suicide. The frenetic and driven behaviour of mania also results in a non-functional individual, but for different reasons. People in this state cannot work effectively, may ruin businesses, and perhaps drive themselves to exhaustion and death.

Affective disorders are more than just extreme points of normal mood-swings. Physiologically, psychologically and behaviourally they appear to be qualitatively different phenomena, and biochemical studies of mood in normal people will probably tell us little about the pathological mood-swings of depression and mania.

There is little disagreement about the symptoms of the affective disorders. However, as with the schizophrenias, there is dispute about the different subtypes of affective disorders. Some investigators stress factors associated with the onset of the disease, activity changes and whether or not the depressive also has manic episodes. These distinctions have given rise to the following suggested dimensions of the affective disorders: endogenous-reactive, retarded-agitated, and monopolar-bipolar.

The purpose of diagnostic categories is to indicate therapy. While there are several appropriate treatments for affective disorders, they are only weakly correlated with diagnostic categories. Thus, on the basis of symptoms presented by a patient, the psychiatrist has little indication of which of a variety of treatments should be prescribed. Since most treatments are now biochemically oriented, some research groups attempt to define subgroups of affective disorders on the basis of the nature of the biochemical pathology and not according to behavioural–emotional symptoms. If it is possible to make objective what is basically a subjective problem, a great therapeutic advance will have been made.

Because of the apparently complementary nature of the symptoms of mania and depression they are frequently described as opposite poles of an affective continuum where "normality" is the mid-point. This has led to biochemical speculation that depression is due to "too little X" and mania is due to "too much X", with normality being the right amount of X (see 11.6). Unfortunately neither of these conceptual conveniences is accurate. Depression and manic symptoms may occur together and, biochemically, affective disorders are too complex to be viewed as being merely too much or too little of anything.

Since manic and depressive symptoms are often present together, it is incorrect to state that mania and depression are opposite poles of an affective continuum.

The typical view that depression represents too little of a particular neurotransmitter, whereas mania represents too much is convenient but almost totally incorrect.

11.12 Genetic factors in the affective disorders

As with the schizophrenias (11.3), there is a tendency for affective disorders to "run in families". A genetic contribution to the affective disorders is also suggested by studies of twins. The high concordance rates for twins raised separately suggest that the disease does not result simply from being raised in an emotionally disturbed environment.

As with schizophrenia, there is a pronounced genetic component to the affective disorders.

A number of studies suggest the following approximate concordance rates for affective disorders: monozygotic twins, 70%; dizygotic twins, 20%; non-twin siblings, 10%. Further, if one parent has a history of affective disorder, the probability of genetically transmitting that liability is 25%. If both parents have histories of affective disorders, the probability of transmission is over 40%. Compare these figures with the overall incidence of depression in most Western countries of 1–5%.

The genetic aspects of affective disorders are sex-dependent. Whereas the overall risk for schizophrenia is approximately the same in both sexes, females are twice as likely as males to develop affective disorders, particularly depression. The somewhat controversial suggestion has been made that the affective disorders, like colour-blindness, may be associated with the X chromosome.

11.13 Are the affective disorders due to a biochemical abnormality?

The same research strategies indicate that schizophrenia and the affective disorders represent primary biochemical abnormalities. Various drugs can induce affective disturbances in normal people, whereas other drugs can alleviate affective symptoms in disturbed patients. Similarly, analysis of body fluids of affectively disturbed people has suggested that something is amiss biochemically. However, the specification of that "something" has been as difficult as in schizophrenia (11.6).

11.14 Biochemical abnormalities in the affective disorders

The direct specification of the biochemical defect in the affective disorders by the analysis of various fluid samples has generated little consistent information.

The content and activity of a wide variety of biological samples from affectively disturbed patients have been investigated with an impressive array of analytical techniques. So far, investigations have provided little solid information about the biochemical pathology which presumably underlies the affective disorders. The disappointing results could be due to at least three factors. First, peripheral samples such as blood and the cerebrospinal fluid do not provide a clear index of the chemical activity of the brain. Second, we may not be looking at the relevant variables, or, if we are, we may be using inappropriate indices of their activity. Third, the diagnostic categories used to correlate various biochemical anomalies may be inappropriate.

Despite the difficulties of this approach, it remains an important area for future research. A rational therapeutic approach can be adopted only when the nature of the underlying pathology has been demonstrated. Advances in the therapy of the major psychoses (schizophrenias and affective disorders) have occurred largely by chance. Concepts such as the "dopamine theory of schizophrenia" or the "noradrenergic theory of depression" have been developed after the fact of successful drug therapies. They have, as yet, done little to improve these therapies or to suggest new ones.

11.15 Biochemically inducing affective disorders

Amphetamine can reliably induce a "model" paranoid schizophrenia (11.5), but it is more difficult to induce affective pathologies pharmacologically.

During the 1950s, it was recognized that some cases of hypertension (high blood pressure) were due partially to excessive peripheral activity of catecholamines. Noradrenalin has a powerful constrictor effect on blood vessels. The therapeutic logic was that by reducing the activity of noradrenalin, hypertension should be reduced correspondingly. The drug *reserpine* causes stored catecholamines to be discharged prematurely, causing a depletion of noradrenalin and the other catecholamines, dopamine and adrenalin. Reserpine had some therapeutic effect on hypertension, but more importantly it had an unexpected adverse psychological side-effect. Approximately 20% of patients given reserpine developed a depression so severe that, in most cases, hospitalization was required and reserpine treatment had to be discontinued. It was later shown that the drug *alpha-methyltyrosine* (which blocks the synthesis of catecholamines) can also induce depression.

Catecholamine depleting drugs can occasionally produce depression.

These results suggest that a reduction in transmission in catecholamine-containing nerve cells can, in a significant number of cases, precipitate depression. The fact that 80% of the cases did not develop depression suggests that the depressions are biochemically diverse and that there are large individual differences in susceptibility to these disorders. The biochemical heterogeneity of the affective disorders is supported by other evidence as well.

Evidence that mania and depression are not simply opposite poles of a mood continuum is also provided by the fact that there is, as yet, no way of inducing mania in normals. While the effects of amphetamine are superficially similar to manic effects, amphetamine has been used, with some success, to treat mania.

11.16 Managing the affective disorders with drugs

Three principal groups of drugs are effective in the management of affective disorders. They are: (1) monoamine oxidase inhibitors; (2) re-uptake blockers; and (3) lithium salts. The therapeutic effects of each group were discovered by accident.

The monoamine oxidase inhibitors and re-uptake blockers are anti-depressants, their main use being for depressive disorders. Lithium is an anti-manic or mood stabilizer, also effective in stabilizing depressive mood-swings. It is used primarily for recurrent, bipolar manic-depressive disorders. Whereas the anti-depressants and mood stabilizers all elevate mood in depressives, they typically have a sedative or mildly depressive effect in normals. Further, stimulant drugs such as cocaine and amphetamine, which tend to elevate mood in normals, generally have little therapeutic effect with depressives. These results suggest that psychiatric depression is not just a greater than normal mood-swing. Pharmacologically and biochemically, depressive disorders appear to be qualitatively distinct phenomena.

Monoamine oxidase (MAO) is the principal enzyme for the destruction of all the monoamine neurotransmitters (nor-adrenalin, adrenalin, dopamine, serotonin). The first medical use of a drug which inhibited MAO was in the treatment of tuberculosis with *iproniazid*. The drug produced an elevation of depressed mood that could not be accounted for by the generally improved health of the patients. Iproniazid and a variety of related compounds are moderately effective anti-depressants.

However, the undesirable side-effects produced by such an indiscriminate enhancement of neurotransmission have greatly restricted their use. Their indiscriminate action has also complicated the determination of which transmitter may be responsible for their therapeutic effectiveness. However, the anti-depressant action of the MAO inhibitors raised the possibility that depression was due to defective (perhaps underactive) transmission in monoaminergic neurons. This approach continues to dominate research in this area.

The monoamine deficiency hypothesis was further supported by the anti-depressant effects of drugs that block the pre-synaptic re-uptake of monoamines. A common example of such a drug is *imipramine*, originally synthesized as a potential anti-schizophrenic agent. It was a poor anti-schizophrenic but a reasonably effective anti-depressant. Because their core molecular structure consists of three rings, imipramine and numerous related drugs are called *tricyclic anti-depressants*. By blocking the re-uptake of monoamines, tricyclic anti-depressants are thought to increase transmitter availability and to enhance synaptic transmission.

Although the original re-uptake blockers produced a fairly indiscriminate increase in monoamine availability (much like the monoamine oxidase inhibitors), some new compounds are more selective. For example, it is now possible to block the re-uptake of either noradrenalin or serotonin selectively. It appears that

Drugs which elevate mood in depressives do not produce a comparable effect in normals. Conversely, mood elevators for normals do not generally work with depressives.

Because of their undesirable side effects, MAO inhibitors are now used only as a last resort in treating depression.

Molecular diagram of the anti-depressant drug imipramine. Its three-ring configuration underlies its classification as a tricyclic anti-depressant.

some patients respond better to noradrenalin re-uptake blockade, whereas others respond better to serotonin re-uptake blockade. These findings provide further evidence for the biochemical heterogeneity of the depressions.

The anti-depressant effect of MAO inhibitors and re-uptake blockers has frequently been interpreted as indicating that depression is due to too little of a particular monoamine. This interpretation is almost certainly incorrect, for a number of reasons. First, fluid analyses have provided little evidence of any such deficit. More importantly, attempts at increasing transmitter levels by administering precursors of the monoamines or by using direct receptor stimulants have been weak and variable in their therapeutic effectiveness. Moreover, cellular level homeostatic processes are generally so efficient that gross changes in neurotransmitter levels rarely occur.

11.17 Shock treatment

Shock treatment is perhaps the oldest and certainly the most infamous therapy for the affective disorders. In spite of the notoriety which it has attracted, electroconvulsive shock (ECS) is still probably the most useful and fast-acting treatment.

ECS has the fastest onset and is arguably the most effective anti-depressant.

Although the induction of seizures by ECS is virtually the only method used today, ECS has a number of interesting antecedents. The vapours of camphor, which can induce massive seizures, were used to treat mania in the late 18th century. In the early 20th century psychiatric patients were "therapeutically" infected with malaria. The coma produced by low blood-sugar levels following large insulin injections was also used to treat affective disorders in the early part of this century. Seizures and coma can also be induced by a variety of drugs, some closely related to camphor. However, the potential lethality and other adverse side effects of such treatments have resulted in their virtual disappearance.

ECS is reasonably safe, painless and arguably the most effective therapy for depression. By pretreating patients with muscle relaxants, the overt muscular spasms that have been extensively dramatized do not occur. The most adverse effects of ECS result from the fear and loathing of the general community. The near-hysterical opposition to ECS by "anti-psychiatry" groups has made many patients unjustifiably frightened of a treatment which may well be beneficial to them. On the other hand, fully justified opposition to ECS followed its extensive misapplication during the 1950s and 1960s. The stigma of the unsuccessful and misguided applications of ECS continues to linger.

The most serious side effects of ECS are generated not by the shock itself but by the fear and loathing of the general community.

The best-documented adverse side effects of ECS is a period

of post-treatment confusion and amnesia for events in the immediate pre-shock period. Some recent experiments restricting ECS to only one side of the brain indicate that the side-effects can be minimized while retaining the full therapeutic effectiveness of ECS. It appears that much of the post-shock confusion and amnesia represents a disruption of verbal processes. Human verbal processes are strongly associated with the left hemisphere. Therefore, if ECS is confined to the right (non-verbal) hemisphere, the adverse side-effects are greatly reduced, and the anti-depressant effect is unchanged.

If ECS is administered to only the right (non-verbal) hemisphere, the post-treatment confusion is minimized while the full therapeutic effectiveness is retained.

Why such a crude and seemingly nonsensical treatment is so effective is the question that remains to be answered. Currently, much research is being directed at the neurochemical changes produced by ECS and the anti-depressant drugs, but a clear explanation is not yet available. This is due partly to the delayed onset of therapeutic effects of the treatments. Anti-depressant treatments produce a variety of relatively specific and immediate changes in several neurotransmitter systems. However, in a clinical context, the therapeutic effects have a time lag ranging from a few days for ECS to a few weeks for anti-depressant drugs. By this time many obvious biochemical effects of the treatments are greatly reduced, or may even disappear. These findings suggest that we have been either looking at the wrong transmitters or using inappropriate indicators of their activity.

11.18 Mood stabilization with lithium

Lithium is most effective in the treatment of manic-depressive disorders.

During the late 1940s, Cade, an Australian researcher, discovered the mood-stabilizing effect of lithium salts. Lithium is one of the most effective and specific psychotherapeutic drugs known. It is particularly effective in treating *bipolar* affective disorders. These disorders are characterized by periods of depression alternating with periods of mania.

As with ECS, it has been difficult to specify how lithium works. Early explanations centred around lithium's similarity to calcium ions, which modulate the synaptic release of neurotransmitters. A new hypothesis is based on results which indicate that lithium produces a biochemical-stabilizing effect closely paralleling its mood-stabilizing effect. Mandel and Knapp have observed that, while lithium has little effect on the normal activity of serotonergic neurons, it does make the neurons resistant to large changes in their activity in either direction. This physiological "buffering" process may account for the findings that lithium seems to allow normal mood-swings, but it inhibits the extreme highs and lows seen in bipolar affective illness. Since the hypothesis deals with only one transmitter (serotonin), it is al-

Although there are a number of hypotheses, the mechanisms of the therapeutic effects of both ECS and lithium are largely unknown.

most certainly an oversimplification. Nevertheless it constitutes a potentially fruitful departure from conventional thinking.

Another unusual hypothesis to account for the therapeutic effects of lithium has been developed by Tissot. He maintains that lithium affects the processes transporting neurotransmitter precursors across the blood–brain barrier. The novel aspect of this hypothesis is that, since the amino acid precursors apparently compete for the same transport medium, lithium would be expected to alter the metabolism of two or more amine-related neurotransmitters. That affective disorders (and other psychiatric problems) are jointly determined by disorder in several neurotransmitter systems, is in accord with contemporary thinking.

When the nature of the biochemical dysfunctions underlying psychiatric problems has been determined, hopefully in the not-too-distant future, we must address ourselves to the next question — how do these abnormalities arise?

Questions

1 Consider some of the limitations of the biological approach to psychiatric problems.
2 Psychoses are rarely cured. Comment.
3 Where would psychiatry be if the term "mental" were to disappear suddenly?
4 What has Hollywood done for (or to) psychiatry?
5 What are the social implications of (and what is the social genesis of) attaching the word "psychotomimetic" to certain drugs?
6 What are some of the problems of inferring brain function from an analysis of body fluids?
7 Discuss the term "major tranquilizer".
8 Schizophrenics have too much dopamine in the brain. Criticize.
9 Depressives are normal people with a low tolerance for suffering. Criticize.
10 Discuss the pharmacotherapy of the affective disorders.
11 Depression is due to there being too little noradrenalin in the brain. Criticize.
12 What are the pros and cons for the therapeutic use of electroconvulsive shock?

Further Readings

Davis, G.C., Bunney, W.E. Jr. Psychopathology and endorphins. *In* E. Costa and M. Trabucchi (Eds) *Neural Peptides and Neuronal Communication.* New York, Raven Press. 1980.

Klawans, H.L., Goetz, C.G. and Perlik, S. Tardive dyskinesia: Review and update. *American Journal of Psychiatry,* 1980, **137**, 900–908.

Lewis, M.E. Biochemical aspects of schizophrenia. *In* M.B.H. Youdin, W. Lovenberg, D.F. Sharman and J.R. Lagnado (Eds). *Essays in Neurochemistry and Neuropharmacology,* Vol. 4. New York, Wiley. 1980.

Murphy, D.L., Campbell, I. and Costa, J.L. Current status of the indoleamine hypothesis of affective disorders. *In* M.A. Lyston, A. Di Mascio and K.F. Killam (Eds). *Psychopharmacology: A Generation of Progress.* New York, Raven Press. 1978.

Schulsinger, F. Biological psychopathology. *Annual Review of Psychology*, 1980, **31**, 583–606.

Kokkinidis, L. and Anisman H. Amphetamine models of paranoid schizophrenia: An overview and elaboration of animal experimentation. *Psychological Bulletin*, 1980, **80**, 551–579.

Zis, A.P. and Goodwin, F.K. Novel antidepressants and the biogenic amine hypothesis of depression. *Archives of General Psychiatry*, 1979, **36**, 1097–1107.

References

Chapter 1

Barker, J.L. Peptides: Roles in neuronal excitability. *Physiological Reviews*, 1976, **56**, 435–452.

Brock, L.G. Coombs, J.S. and Eccles, J.C. The recording of potentials from motoneurons with an intracellular electrode. *Journal of Physiology*, 1952, **117**, 431–460.

Burnstock, G. Do some nerve cells release more than one transmitter. *Neuroscience*, 1976, **1**, 239–248.

Cooper, J.R. Bloom, F.E. and Roth, R.H. *The Biochemical Basis of Neuropharmacology*. New York, Oxford University Press. 1978.

de Jong, R.H. Minireview: Neural blockade by local anesthetics. *Life Sciences*, 1977, **20**, 915–920.

Dismukes, R.K. New concepts of molecular communication among neurons. *The Behavioural and Brain Sciences*, 1979, **2**, 409–448.

Eccles, J.C. *The Physiology of Synapses*. Berlin, Springer-Verlag. 1974.

Eccles, J.C. *The Physiology of Nerve Cells*. Baltimore, Md., Johns Hopkins Press. 1957.

Eisinger, J. Biochemistry and measurement of environmental lead intoxication. *Quarterly Reviews of Biophysics*, 1978, **11**, 439–466.

Henn, F.A. Neurotransmission and glial cells: A functional relationship? *Journal of Neuroscience Research*, 1976, **2**, 271–282.

Hökfelt, T., Lundberg, J.M., Schultzberg, M., Johansson, O., Ljungdahl, A. and Rehfeld, J. Coexistence of peptides and putative transmitters in neurons. *In* E. Costa and M. Trabucchi (Eds) *Neural Peptides and Neuronal Communication*. New York, Raven Press. 1980.

Hubel, D.H. The brain. *Scientific American*, 1979, **241** (3), 38–47.

Hughes, J. Isolation of an endogenous compound from the brain with pharmacological properties similar to morphine. *Brain Research*, 1975, **88**, 295–308.

Hughes, J., Smith, T.W., Kosterlitz, H.W., Fothergill, L.A., Morgan, B.A. and Morris, H.R. Identification of two related pentapeptides from the brain with potent opiate agonist activity. *Nature*, 1975, **258**, 577–579.

Iversen, S.D. and Iversen, L.L. Chemical pathways in the brain. *In* M. Gazzaniga and C. Blakemore (Eds) *Handbook of Psychobiology*. New York, Academic Press, 1975.

Kurland, L.T., Faro, S. and Siedler, H. Minamata disease. The outbreak of a neurologic disorder in Minamata, Japan, and its relationship to the ingestion of seafood contaminated by mercuric compounds. *World Neurology*, 1960, **1**, 370–395.

Mervis, R. Structural alterations in neurons of aged canine neocortex: A Golgi study. *Experimental Neurology*, 1978, **62**, 417–432.

Mulder, A.H. and Snyder, S.H. Putative central neurotransmitters. *In* W.H. Gespin (Ed) *Molecular and Functional Neurobiology*. Amsterdam, Elsevier. 1976.

Reuhl, K.R. and Chang, L.W. Effects of methymercury on the development of the nervous system: A review. *Neurotoxicology*, 1979, **1**, 21–55.

Schmitt, F.O., Dev, P. and Smith, B.H. Electronic processing of information by brain cells. *Science*, 1976, **193**, 114–120.

Smith, D.O. Reduced capabilities of synaptic transmission in aged rats. *Experimental Neurology*. 1979, **66**, 650–666.

Snyder, S.H. Brain peptides as neurotransmitters. *Science*, 1980. **209**, 976–983.

Stevens, C.F. The neuron. *Scientific American*, 1979, **241** (3), 48–59.

Sturrock, R.R. A quantitative lifespan study of changes in cell number, cell division and cell death in various regions of the mouse forebrain. *Neuropathology and Applied Neurobiology*, 1979, **5**, 433–456.

Chapter 2

Bures, J., Petran, M. and Zachar, J. *Electrophysiological Methods in Biological Research*. New York, Academic Press. 1967.

Falck, B., Hillarp, N.-A., Thieme, G. and Torp, A. Fluorescence of catecholamines and related compounds condensed with formaldehyde. *Journal of Histochemistry and Cytochemistry*, 1962, **10**, 348–354.

Fuxe, K., Hökfelt, T. and Ungerstedt, V. Morphological and functional aspects of central monoamine neurons. *International Review of Neurobiology*, 1970, **13**, 93–126.

Kumar, R. Animal models of psychiatric disorders. *In* H.M. van Praag (Ed.) *Handbook of Biological Psychiatry*. New York, Marcel Dekker. 1979.

Raichle, M. Cerebral blood flow and metabolism in man: Past, present and future. *Trends in Neurosciences*, 1980, **3**, VI-X.

Robertson, R.T. *Neuroanatomical Research Techniques*. New York, Academic Press. 1978.

Sokoloff, L., Reivich, M., Kennedy, C., Des Rosiers, M.H., Patlak, C.S., Pettigrew, K.D., Sakurada, O. and Shinohara, M. The (^{14}C) deoxyglucose method for the measurement of local cerebral glucose utilization: Theory, procedure and normal values in the conscious and anesthetized albino rat. *Journal of Neurochemistry*, 1977, **28**, 897–917.

Thompson, R.F. and Patterson, M.M. *Bioelectric Recording Techniques* (3 vols). New York, Academic Press. 1973.

Chapter 3

Brodal, A. *Neurological Anatomy*, 2nd ed. New York, Oxford University Press. 1969.

Jerison, H.J. Paleoneurology and the evolution of mind. *Scientific American*, 1976, **234**, 90–101.

Krieg, W.J.S. *Functional Neuroanatomy*. New York, Blakiston. 1942.

Mettler, F.A. and Mettler, C.C. The effects of striatal injury. *Brain*, 1942, **65**, 242–255.

Myers, R.D. Psychopharmacology of alcohol. *Annual Review of Pharmacology and Toxicology*. 1978, **18**, 125–144.

Nauta, W.J.H. and Feirtag, M. The organization of the brain. *Scientific American*, 1979, **241**, (3), 78–105.

Papez, J.W. A proposed mechanism of emotion. *Archives of Neurology and Psychiatry*. 1937, **38**, 725–744.

Schally, A.V., Kastin, A.J. and Arimura, A. Hypothalamic hormones: The link between brain and body. *American Scientist*, 1977, **65**, 712–719.

van der Bercken, J.H.L. and Cools, A.R. Role of the neostriatum in the initiation, continuation and termination of behavior. *Applied Neurophysiology*, 1979, **42**, 106–108.

Yahr, M.D. (Ed.) *The Basal Ganglia*. New York, Raven Press. 1976.

Chapter 4

Bannister, R. *Brain's Clinical Neurology*, 5th ed. New York, Oxford University Press. 1978.

Bjorklund, A. and Stenevi, U. Regeneration of monoaminergic and cholinergic neurons in the mammalian central nervous system. *Physiological Reviews,* 1979, **59**, 62–100.

Bogen, J.E. and Bogen, G.M. Wernicke's region — Where is it? *Annals of the New York Academy of Sciences,* 1976, **280**, 834–843.

Bogen, J.E. and Vogel, P.J. Cerebral commissurotomy in man: Preliminary case report. *Bulletin of the Los Angeles Neurological Society,* 1962, **27**, 169–172.

Brown, J. *Aphasia, Apraxia and Agnosia.* Springfield, Ill., C.C. Thomas. 1972.

Evarts, E.V. Brain mechanisms of movement. *Scientific American,* 1979, **241** (3), 146–156.

Gazzaniga, M.S. *The Bisected Brain.* New York, Appleton–Century–Crofts. 1970.

Gazzaniga, M.S. Review of the split brain. *Journal of Neurology,* 1975, **209**, 75–79.

Gazzaniga, M.S., Bogen, J.E. and Sperry, R.W. Observations on visual perception after disconnexion of the cerebral hemispheres in man. *Brain,* 1965, **88**, 221–236.

Geschwind, N. The organisation of language and the brain. *Science,* 1970, **170**, 940–944.

Geschwind, N. The Apraxias: Neural mechanisms of disorders of learned movement. *American Scientist,* 1975, **63**, 188–195.

Hardyck, C. and Petrinovich, L.F. Left-handedness. *Psychological Bulletin,* 1977, **84**, 385–404.

Jacobsen, C.F. Studies of cerebral function in primates. *Comparative Psychology Monographs,* 1936, **13**, 1–68.

Jacobson, M. *Developmental Neurobiology.* New York, Plenum. 1978.

Jorm, A.F. The cognitive and neurological basis of developmental dyslexia: A theoretical framework and review. *Cognition,* 1979, **7**, 19–33.

LeVere, T.E. Neural stability, sparing and behavioral recovery following brain damage. *Psychological Review,* 1975, **82**, 344–358.

LeVere, T.E., Davis, N. and Gonder, L. Recovery of function after brain damage: Toward understanding the deficit. *Physiological Psychology,* 1979, **7**, 317–326.

Luria, A.R. *Higher Cortical Functions in Man.* New York, Basic Books, 1966.

Luria, A.R. *The Working Brain.* New York, Penguin. 1973.

Luria, A.R. and Hutton, J.T. A modern assessment of the basic forms of aphasia. *Brain and Language,* 1977, **4**, 129–151.

Mateer, C. and Kimura, D. Impairment of nonverbal oral movements in aphasia. *Brain and Language,* 1977, **4**, 262–272.

Milner, B. Some effects of frontal lobectomy in man. *In* J.M. Warren and K. Akert (Eds) *The Frontal Granular Cortex and Behavior.* New York, McGraw-Hill. 1964.

Noback, C.R. and Demarest, R.J. *The Nervous System.* New York, McGraw-Hill. 1977.

Passingham, R.E. Brain size and intelligence in man. *Brain Behavior and Evolution,* 1979, **16**, 253–270.

Penfield, W. and Boldrey, E. Somatic motor and sensory representation in the cerebral cortex as studied by electrical stimulation. *Brain,* 1958, **60**, 389–443.

Penfield, W. and Jasper, H.H. *Epilepsy and the Functional Anatomy of the Human Brain.* Boston, Little Brown. 1954.

Penfield, W. and Rasmussen, T. *The Cerebral Cortex of Man: A Clinical Study of Localization of Function.* New York, Crowell-Collier and Macmillan. 1950.

Penfield, W. and Roberts, L. *Speech and Brain Mechanisms.* Princeton, N.J., Princeton University Press. 1959.

Pribram, K.H. The primate frontal cortex — Executive of the brain. *In* K.H. Pribram and A.R. Luria (Eds) *Psychophysiology of the Frontal Lobes.* New York, Academic Press. 1974.

Prince, D.A. Neurophysiology of epilepsy. *Annual Review of Neuroscience,* 1978, **1**, 395–415.

Raisman, G. What hope for repair of the brain? *Annals of neurology,* 1978, **3**, 101–106.

Richardson, D.E. Brain stimulation for pain control. *IEEE Transactions on Biomedical Engineering,* 1976, **BME-23**, 304–306.

Sperry, R.W. Cerebral organization and behaviour. *Science,* 1961, **133**, 1749–1757.

Sperry, R.W. Lateral specialisation in the surgically separated hemispheres. *In* F.O. Schmitt and F.G. Worden (Eds) *The Neurosciences: Third Study Program.* Cambridge, Mass., M.I.T. Press. 1974.

Sperry, R.W., Stamm, J.S. and Miner, N. Relearning tests for interocular transfer following division of optic chiasma and corpus callosum in cats. *Journal of Comparative and Physiological Psychology,* 1956, **49**, 529–533.

Warren, S. M. and Nonneman, A.J. The search for cerebral dominance in monkeys. *Annals of the New York Academy of Sciences,* 1976, **280**, 732–744.

Witelson, S. F. Sex and the single hemisphere: Specialisation of the right hemisphere for spatial processing. *Science,* 1976, **193**, 425–427.

Chapter 5

Aitkin, L.M. The auditory midbrain. *Trends in Neurosciences,* 1979, **2**, 308–310.

Albe-Fessard, D. and Fessard, A. Recent advances on the neurophysiological bases of pain sensation. *Acta neurobiologica Experimentalis,* 1976, **35**, 715–740.

Amoore, J.E. Stereochemical and vibrational theories of odour. *Nature,* 1971, **233**, 270–271.

Amoore, S.E. Specific anosmia and the concept of primary odors. *Chemical Senses and Flavor,* 1977, **2**, 267–278.

Arvidson, K. and Friberg, U. Human taste: Response and taste bud number in fungiform papillae. *Science,* 1980, **209**, 807–808.

Barlow, H.B. and Hill, R.M. Evidence for a physiological explanation of the waterfall phenomenon and figural after-effects. *Nature,* 1963, **200**, 1345–1347.

Barlow, H.B. and Levick, W.R. Threshold setting by the surround of cat retinal ganglion cells. *Journal of Physiology,* 1976, **259**, 737–757.

Blakemore, C. Developmental factors in the formation of feature-extracting neurons. *In* F.O. Schmitt and F.G. Worden (Eds) *The Neurosciences: Third Study Program,* Cambridge, Mass., M.I.T. Press. 1974.

Blakemore, C. Maturation and modification in the developing visual system. *In* R. Held, H.W. Leibowitz and H.-L. Teuber (Eds) *Handbook of Sensory Physiology,* Vol.3. *Perception.* pp.377–436. Berlin, Springer. 1978.

Blakemore, C. and Campbell, F.W. On the existence in the human visual system of neurons selectively sensitive to the orientation and size of retinal images. *Journal of Physiology,* 1969, **203**, 237–260.

Blakemore, C. and Cooper, G.F. Development of the brain depends on the visual environment. *Nature,* 1970, **228**, 477–478.

Brugge, J.F. and Merzenich, M.M. Patterns of activity of single neurons of the auditory cortex in monkey. *In* A.R. Møller, (Ed.) *Basic Mechanisms in Hearing.* New York, Academic Press. 1973.

Cardello, A.V. Taste quality changes as a function of salt concentration in single human taste papillae. *Chemical Senses and Flavor,* 1979, **4**, 1–13.

Cornsweet, T.N. *Visual Perception.* New York, Academic Press. 1970.

Dallos, P. *The Auditory Periphery: Biophysics and Physiology.* New York, Academic Press. 1973.

De Valois, R.L. and Jacobs, G.H. Primate color vision. *Science,* 1968, **162**, 533–540.

De Valois, R.L. Abramov, I. and Mead, W.R. Single cell analysis of wavelength discrimination at the lateral geniculate nucleus in the macagne. *Journal of Neurophysiology,* 1967, **30**, 415–433.

Evans, E.F. Neural processes for the detection of acoustic patterns and for sound localisation. *In* F.O. Schmitt and F.G. Worden (Eds) *The Neurosciences: Third Study Program.* Cambridge, Mass., M.I.T. Press. 1974.

Green, D.M. *An Introduction to Hearing.* Hillsdale, N.J., Lawrence Erlbaum. 1976.

Gulick, W.L. *Hearing: Physiology and Psychophysics.* New York, Oxford University Press. 1971.

Hartline, H.K. and Ratliff, F. Inhibitory interaction of receptor units in the eye of *Limulus. Journal of General Physiology,* 1957, **40**, 357–376.

Hering, E. *Zur Lehre vom Lichtsinn.* Wien, Carl Gerold's Sohn. 1878.

Hirsch, H.V.B. and Spinelli, D.N. Visual experience modifies distribution of horizontally and vertically oriented receptive fields in cats. *Science,* 1970, **168**, 869–871.

Houpt, K.A. and Houpt, T.R. Comparative aspects of the ontogeny of taste. *Chemical Senses and Flavor,* 1976, **2**, 219-228.

Hubel, D.H. and Wiesel, T.N. Integrative action in the cat's lateral geniculate body. *Journal of Physiology,* 1961, **155**, 385–398.

Hubel, D.H. and Wiesel, T.N. Receptive fields of single neurones in the cat's striate cortex. *Journal of Physiology,* 1959, **148**, 574–591.

Hubel, D.H. and Wiesel, T.N. Receptive fields, binocular interaction and functional architecture in the cat's visual cortex. *Journal of Physiology,* 1962, **160**, 106–154.

Kiang, N.Y.-S. Processing of speech by the auditory nervous system. *Journal of the Acoustical Society of America.* 1980. **68**, 830–835.

Kiang, N.Y.-S. and Moxon, E.C. Tails of tuning curves of auditory nerve fibers. *Journal of the Acoustical Society of America.* 1974, **55**, 620–630.

Kiang, N.Y.-S., Watanabe, T., Thomas, E.C. and Clark, L.F. *Discharge Patterns of Single Fibers in the Cat's Auditory Nerve,* Cambridge, Mass., M.I.T. Press, 1965.

Kuffler, S.W. Discharge patterns and functional organization of mammalian retina. *Journal of Neurophysiology,* 1953, **16**, 37–68.

Lennie, P. Parallel visual pathways: a review. *Vision Research,* 1980, **20**, 561–594.

Lian, A. Müller's doctrine of specific nerve energies. *Scandanavian Journal of Psychology,* 1976, **17**, 133–141.

Mathews, D.F. Rat olfactory nerve responses to odor. *Chemical Senses and Flavor,* 1974, **1**, 69–76.

McBurney, D.H. Are there primary tastes for man? *Chemical Senses and Flavor,* 1974, **1**, 17–28.

Melzack, R.R. *The Puzzle of Pain.* New York, Basic Books. 1973.

Merzenich, M.M., Michelson, R.P., Pettit, C.R., Schindler, R.A. and Reid, M. Neural encoding of sound sensations evoked by electrical stimulation of the acoustic nerve. *Annals of Otology, Rhinology and Laryngology,* 1973, **82**, 1–18.

Mitchell, D.E. Freeman, R.D. Millodot, M., and Haegerstrom, G. Meridional amblyopia: Evidence for modification of the human visual system by early experience. *Vision Research,* 1973, **13**, 535–558.

Moulton, D.G. Spatial patterning of response to odors in the peripheral olfactory system. *Physiological Reviews,* 1976, **56**, 578–593.

Mountcastle, V.B. Brain mechanisms for directed attention. *Journal of the Royal Society of Medicine,* 1978, **71**, 14–28.

Müller, J. *Handbuch der Physiologie der Menschen.* Coblenz, Verlag von J. Holscher. 1838.

Nathan, P.W. The gate-control theory of pain. A critical review. *Brain,* 1976, **99**, 123–158.

Nathan, P. W. Pain. *British Medical Bulletin,* 1977, **33**, 149–156.

Naunton, R.F. *The Vestibular System.* New York, Academic Press. 1975.

Pfaffmann, C. Gustatory nerve impulses in rat, cat and rabbit. *Journal of Neurophysiology,* 1955, **18**, 429–440.

Pöppel, E., Held, R. and Frost, D. Residual visual function after brain wounds involving the central visual pathways in man. *Nature,* 1973, **243**, 295–296.

Rodieck, R.W. *The Vertebrate Retina.* San Francisco, Ca., W.H. Freeman. 1973.

Rushton, W.A. H. Kinetics of cone pigments measured objectively on the living human fovea. *Annals of the New York Academy of Sciences,* 1958, **74**, 291–304.

Sanders, M.D., Warrington, E.K., Marshall, J. and Weiskrantz, L. "Blindsight": vision in a field defect. *The Lancet,* 1974 (April 20), 707–708.

Schiffman, S.S. and Erickson, R. P. The issue of primary taste versus a taste continuum. *Neuroscience and Biobehavioral Reviews,* 1980, **4**, 109–117.

Stone, J. Dreher, B. and Leventhal, A. Hierarchical and parallel mechanisms in the organization of visual cortex. *Brain Research Reviews,* 1979, **1**, 345–394.

Tonndorf, J. Cochlear prostheses. *Annals of Otology, Rhinology and Laryngology* 1977, **86**, (Supplement 44), 1–20.

von Békésy, G. *Experiments in Hearing.* New York, McGraw-Hill, 1960.

von Békésy, G. Duplexity theory of taste. *Science,* 1964, **145**, 834–835.

von Békésy, G. Taste theories and the chemical stimulation of single papillae. *Journal of Applied Physiology,* 1966, **21**, 1–9.

von Békésy, G. *Sensory Inhibition.* Princeton, Princeton University Press, 1967.

von Frey, M. and Kiesow, F. Veber die Function der Tastkörperchen. *Zeitschrift für Psychologie,* 1899, **20**, 126–163.

von Helmholtz, H.L.F. *Treatise on Physiological Optics.* J.P.C. Southall (translator) 1924. New York, Dover. 1962.

von Kries, J. Die Gesichtsempfindungen. *In* W. Nagel (Ed.) *Handbuch der Physiologie des Menschens,* Vol. 3. Braunschweig, Viegweg. 1905.

Wilson, V.J. and Melvill Jones, G. *Mammalian Vestibular Physiology.* New York, Plenum. 1979.

Young, T. On the theory of light and colours. In *Lectures in Natural Philosophy,* printed for Joseph Johnson. London, Savage. 1807.

Zeki, S. The representation of colours in the cerebral cortex. *Nature,* 1980, **284**, 412–418.

Chapter 6

Akerstedt, T. and Fröberg, J.E. Sleep and stressor exposure in relation to circadian rhythms in catecholamine excretion. *Biological Psychology*, 1979, **8**, 69–80.

Allison, T. and Cicchetti, D.V. Sleep in mammals: Ecological and constitutional correlates. *Science*, 1976, **194**, 732–734.

Dement, W., Holman, R.B. and Guilleminault, C. Neurochemical and neuropharmacological foundations of the sleep disorders. *Psychopharmacology Communications*, 1976, **2**, 77–90.

Hartmann, E. and Brewer, V. When is more or less sleep required? A study of variable sleepers. *Comprehensive Psychiatry*, 1976, **17**, 275–284.

Jouvet, M. Cholinergic mechanisms and sleep. *In* P.G. Wasser (Ed.) *Cholinergic Mechanisms.* New York, Raven Press. 1975.

Laing, G.C. and Salzarulo P. (Eds) *Experimental Study of Human Sleep: Methodological Problems.* Amsterdam, Elsevier. 1975.

Lee, S.G.M. and Mayes, A.R. *Dreams and Dreaming.* London, Penguin. 1973.

Pappenheimer, J.R. The sleep factor. *Scientific American*, 1976, **235** (2), 24–29.

Reiter, R.J. Pineal interaction with the central nervous system. *Waking and Sleeping*, 1977, **1**, 253–258.

Svendses, K. Sleep deprivation therapy in depression. *Acta Psychiatrica Scandinavica*, 1976, **54**, 184–192.

Vogel, G.W. A review of REM sleep deprivation. *Archives of General Psychiatry*, 1975, **32**, 749–776.

Vogel, G.W., Vogel, F., McAbee, R.S. and Thurmond, A.J. Improvement of depression by REM sleep deprivation. *Archives of General Psychiatry*, 1980, **37**, 247–253.

Webb, P. and Hiestand, M. Sleep metabolism and age. *Journal of Applied Physiology*, 1975, **38**, 257–262.

Chapter 7

Blass, E.M. and Hall, W.G. Drinking termination: Interactions among hydrational, orogastric and behavioral controls in rats. *Psychological Review*, 1976, **83**, 356–374.

Booth, D.A. Satiety and appetite are conditioned reactions. *Psychosomatic Medicine*, 1977, **39**, 76–81.

Faust, I.M., Johnson, P.R., Stern, J.S. and Hirsch, J. Diet-induced adipocyte number increase in adult rats: A new model of obesity. *American Journal of Physiology*, 1978, **235**, 279–286.

Friedman, M.I. and Stricker, G.M. The physiological psychology of hunger: A physiological perspective. *Psychological Review*, 1976, **83**, 409–431.

Griffiths, M. and Payne, P.R. Energy expenditure in small children of obese and non-obese parents. *Nature*, 1976, **260**, 698–700.

Hill, W., Castonguay, T.W. and Collier, G.H. Taste or diet balancing? *Physiology and Behavior*, 1980, **24**, 765–767.

Keesey, R.E. and Powley, T.L. Hypothalamic regulation of body weight. *American Scientist*, 1975, **63**, 558–565.

Leon, G.R. and Roth, L. Obesity: Psychological causes, correlations and speculations. *Psychological Bulletin*, 1977, **87**, 117–139.

Martin, C.R. *Textbook of Endocrine Physiology.* Baltimore, Md., Williams & Wilkins, 1976.

Moore, R., Grant, A.M., Howard, A.N. and Mills, I.H. Treatment of obesity with triidothyronine and a very-low-calorie liquid formula diet. *Lancet*, 1980, **2**, 223–226.

Myers, R.D., Simpson, C.W., Higgins, D., Natterman, R.A., Rice, J.C., Redgrave, P., and Metcalf, G. Hypothalamic Na^+ and Ca^{2+} ions and temperature set-point: New mechanisms of action of a central or peripheral thermal challenge and intrahypothalamic 5HT, NE, PGE_1 and pyrogen. *Brain Research Bulletin*, 1976, **1**, 301–327.

Rowland, N.E. and Antelman, S.M. Stress-induced hyperphagia and obesity in rats: A possible model for understanding human obesity. *Science*, 1976, **191**, 310–312.

Sclafani, A. and Springer, D. Dietary obesity in adult rats: Similarities to hypothalamic and human obesity syndromes. *Physiology and Behavior*, 1976, **17**, 461–471.

Spiegel, T.A. and Jordon, H.A. Effects of simultaneous oral-intragastric ingestion on meal patterns and satiety in humans. *Journal of Comparative and Physiological Psychology*, 1978, **92**, 1333–1341.

Stricker, G.M., Bradshaw, W.G. and McDonald, R.H. Jr. The renin–angiotensin system and thirst: A re-evaluation. *Science*, 1976, **194**, 1169–1171.

Tepperman, J. *Metabolic and Endocrine Physiology.* Chicago, Ill., Year Book Medical Publishers Inc, 1962.

Trayhurn, P., Thurlby, P.L. and James, W.P.T. Thermogenic defect in pre-obese ob/ob mice. *Nature*, 1977, **266**, 60–62.

Wooley, S.C. and Wooley, O.W. Salivation to the sight and thought of food: A new measure of appetite. *Psychosomatic Medicine*, 1973, **35**, 136–142.

Chapter 8

Atrens, D.M. and Becker, F.T. Cardiovascular responses and lateral hypothalamic self-stimulation: Anatomical differentiation and functional significance. *Brain Research*, 1977, **129**, 29–36.

Atrens, D.M., Ungerstedt, U. and Ljungberg, T. Specific inhibition of hypothalamic self-stimulation by selective re-uptake blockade of either 5-hydroxytryptamine or noradrenalin. *Psychopharmacology*, 1977, **52**, 177–180.

Bishop, M.P., Elder, S.T. and Heath, R.G. Intracranial self-stimulation in man. *Science*, 1963, **140**, 394–396.

Cytawa, J., Jurkowlaniec, E. and Bialowas, J. Positive reinforcement produced by noradrenergic stimulation of the hypothalamus in rats. *Physiology and Behavior*, 1980, **25**, 615–619.

Franklin, K.B.J. and Herberg, L.J. Noncontingent displacement of catecholamines by intraventricular tyramine: Biphasic dose-response effects on self-stimulation. *Neuropharmacology*, 1977, **16**, 53–55.

German, D.C. and Bowden, D.M. Catecholamine systems as the neural substrate for intracranial self-stimulation: A hypothesis. *Brain Research*, 1974, **73**, 381–419.

Hoebel, B.G. Hypothalamic self-stimulation and stimulation escape in relation to feeding and mating. *Federation Proceedings*, 1979, **38**, 2454–2461.

Chapter 9

Bandler, R.J. and Flynn, J.P. Neural Pathways from thalamus in the regulation of aggressive behavior. *Science*, 1974, **183**, 96–99.

Frederickson, R.C.A. and Norris, F.H. Enkephalin-induced depression of single neurons in brain areas with opiate receptors — antagonism by naloxone. *Science*, 1976, **194**, 440–442.

Leib, W., Taylor, W.W. and Stroebel, C.S. Alpha biofeedback: Fact or artifact? *Psychophysiology*, 1976, **13**, 541–545.

Navaco, R.W. The functions and regulation of the arousal of anger. *American Journal of Psychiatry*, 1976, **133**, 1124–1128.

Paxinos, G., Burt, J., Atrens, D.M. and Jackson, D.M. 5-Hydroxytryptamine depletion with parachlorophenylalanine: Effects on eating, drinking, irritability, muricide and copulation. *Pharmacology Biochemistry and Behavior*, 1977, **6**, 439–447.

Rapport, S.I. Opening of the blood–brain barrier by acute hypertension. *Experimental Neurology*, 1976, **52**, 467–479.

Reis, D.J. Central neurotransmitters in aggression. *In* A.R.N.M.D. *Aggression* (Research Publication 52), Association for Research in Nervous and Mental Disease, U.S.A., 1974.

Stein, M., Schiavi, R.C. and Cameriso, M. Influence of brain and behavior on the immune system. *Science*, 1976, **191**, 435–440.

Thornton, E.W. and Hagan, P.J. A failure to explain the effects of false heart-rate feedback on affect induced by changes in physiological response. *British Journal of Psychology*, 1976, **67**, 359–365.

Chapter 10

Fuld, P.A. Storage, retention, and retrieval in Korsakoff's Syndrome. *Neuropsychologia*, 1976, **14**, 225–236.

Gaito, J. Molecular psychobiology of memory: its appearance, contributions and decline. *Physiological Psychology*, 1976, **4**, 476–484.

Gibbs, M.E. Modulation of cycloheximide-resistant memory by sympathomimetic agents. *Pharmacology, Biochemistry and Behavior*, 1976, **4**, 703–707.

Huston, J.P. Learning in the thalamic rat. *In* T.L. Frigyesi, (Ed.) *Subcortical Mechanisms and Sensorimotor Activities*. Hans Huber, Bern. 1975.

Kesner, R.P., Priano, D.J. and De Witt, J.R. Time dependent disruption of morphine tolerance by electro-convulsive shock and frontal cortical stimulation. *Science*, 1976, **194**, 1079–1081.

Marx, S.L. Learning and Behavior (1): Effects of pituitary hormones. *Science*, 1975, **190**, 367–370.

Marx, S.L. Learning and Behavior (II): The hypothalamic peptides. *Science*, 1975, **190**, 544–545.

Penfield, W. and Mathieson, G. Memory. Autopsy findings and comments on the role of hippocampus in experiential recall. *Archives of Neurology*, 1974, **31**, 145–154.

Ungar, G. Molecular coding of memory. *Life Sciences*, 1974, **14**, 595–604.

Wallace, P. Complex environments: Effects on brain development. *Science*, 1974, **185**, 1035–1037.

Wallace, P. Neurochemistry: Unravelling the mechanism of memory. *Science*, 1975, **190**, 1076–1078.

Chapter 11

Arget, J., Frey, R., Lohsneyer, B. and Zerbin-Rubin, E. Bipolar manic-depressive psychosis: Results of a genetic investigation. *Human Genetics*, 1980, **55**, 237–254.

Andren, H.E. Treatment or mistreatment in psychiatry (Observations on electroconvulsive therapy). *Diseases of the Nervous System*, 1976, **37**, 605–609.

Bloom, F., Segal, D., Ling, N. and Guillemin, R. Endorphins: Profound behavioral effects in rats suggest new etiological factors in mental illnes. *Science*, 1976, **194**, 630–632.

Burt, D.R., Creese, I. and Snyder, S.H. Anti-schizophrenic drugs: Chronic treatment elevates dopamine receptor binding in brain. *Science*, 1977, **196**, 326–327.

Carpenter, W.T. Current diagnostic concepts in schizophrenia. *American Journal of Psychiatry*, 1976, **133**, 172–177.

Cochran, E., Robins, E. and Grote, S. Regional serotonin levels in brain: A comparison of depressive suicides and alcoholic suicides with controls. *Biological Psychiatry*, 1976, **11**, 283–294.

Cools, A.R. and van Rossum, J.M. Multiple receptors in behavior regulation: Concept of dopamine-E and dopamine-I receptors. *Life Sciences*, 1980, **27**, 1237–1253.

Costello, C.G. Electroconvulsive therapy: Is further investigation necessary? *Canadian Psychiatric Association Journal*, 1976, **21**, 61–67.

Crow, T.J., Deakin, J.F.W., Johnstone, E.C. and Longden, A. Dopamine and schizophrenia. *The Lancet*, 1976, 563–566.

Davis, J.M. Recent developments in the drug treatment of schizophrenia. *American Journal of Psychiatry*, 1976, **133**, 208–214.

Maas, S.W. Biogenic amines and depression. Biochemical and pharmacological separation of two types of depression. *Archives of General Psychiatry*, 1975, **32**, 1357–1361.

Mandell, A.J. and Knapp, S. A neurobiological model for the symmetrical prophylactic action of lithium in bipolar affective disorder. *Pharmakopsychiatrie Neuro-Psychopharmakologie*, 1976, **9**, 116–126.

Mendels, J. Lithium in the treatment of depression. *American Journal of Psychiatry*, 1976, **133**, 373–378.

Modigh, K. Long term effects of electroconvulsive shock therapy on synthesis turnover and uptake of brain monoamines, *Psychopharmacology*, 1976, **49**, 179–185.

Olsen, R.W., Reisine, T.D. and Yamamura, H.I. Neurotransmitter receptors — Biochemistry and alterations in neuropsychiatric disorders. *Life Sciences*, 1980, **27**, 801–808.

Post, R.M., Kotin, J. and Goodwin, F.K. Effects of sleep deprivation on mood and central amine metabolism in depressed patients. *Archives of General Psychiatry*, 1976, **33**, 627–632.

Shevitz, S.A. Psychosurgery: Some current observation. *American Journal of Psychiatry*, 1976, **133**, 266–270.

Snyder, S.H. The dopamine hypothesis of schizophrenia: Focus on the dopamine receptor. *American Journal of Psychiatry*, 1976, **133**, 197–202.

Tissot, R. The common pathophysiology of monoaminergic psychoses: A new hypothesis. *Neuropsychobiology*, 1975, **1**, 243–260.

Van Praag, H.M. and Korf, S. Central monoamine deficiency in depressions: Causative or secondary phenomenon? *Pharmakopychiatrie Neuro-Psychopharmakologie*, 1975, **8**, 322–326.

Index

3 4 5 6 7 8 9 0 1
B C D E F G H I J